History and Symptoms:
The Eye Examination

With fictional characters to aid history-taking

Jason Searle BSc(Hons) MCOptom Prof Cert Glauc.

Copyright © 2024 by Jason Searle
All rights reserved.
No part of this book may be reproduced, distributed, or transmitted in any form or by any means, including photocopying, recording, or other electronic or mechanical methods, without the prior written permission of the publisher, except in the case of brief quotations embodied in critical reviews and certain other non-commercial uses permitted by copyright law. For permissions requests, write to the publisher, addressed "Attention: Permissions Coordinator," at the email address below:
jason@theeyecareadvocate.co.uk
ISBN 9798303183766
First Printed, 2024

ANTI-PIRACY NOTICE

Dear fellow optometrist,

Thank you for purchasing this copy of "*History and Symptoms: The Eye Examination*".

As a valued member of the optometric community, you are entrusted with upholding the highest standards of professional integrity. It is imperative to remember that as regulated professionals, your actions are governed by the General Optical Council. Adherence to these regulations is not only a reflection of your commitment to the profession but also a legal obligation.

This Study Guide is a product of diligent work and dedication, aimed at enhancing the knowledge and skills of students and optometric professionals like yourself. By respecting this anti-piracy notice, you contribute to a culture of honesty and support the ongoing efforts to provide quality educational materials.

Please be aware that unauthorised copying, distribution, or use of this material is not only unlawful but also considered an act of dishonesty—a serious breach of the ethical code set forth by the General Optical Council. Such actions undermine the trust placed in you by the public and your peers. Whilst this Study Guide is designed to be used in group study, please respect my wishes to not distribute additional copies of this work without my explicit consent.

Furthermore, the proceeds from this publication are reinvested into future projects and the creation of additional Study Guides. Your purchase ensures that The Eye Care Advocate Website can continue to offer the bulk of its content for free, benefiting the wider community and fostering the growth of our field.

Thank you for your support and for standing against piracy.

Respectfully,

J. Searle

Jason Searle

Contents

Anti-Piracy Notice — 3

Introduction — 5

Why is taking a case history important? — 7

How to effectively take a case history — 9

What to include on a primary care case history — 18

Case Study Scripts — 29

Case Study Selection 1: Routine Eye Examinations — 32

Case Study Selection 2: Visual Concerns — 53

Case Study Selection 3: Ocular Pain and Discomfort — 88

Closing Notes — 110

Further Reading — 111

About the Author — 112

Acknowledgements — 113

Introduction

Welcome to "*History & Symptoms: The Eye Examination*", an in-depth book created to help guide the way students and professionals approach the crucial skill of gathering patient histories. Whether you're a seasoned healthcare practitioner, an aspiring optometrist, or someone helping students on their way to qualification, this resource aims to enhance the art of history-taking through engaging fictional case studies.

Patient histories are the foundation of effective healthcare, guiding diagnosis and treatment. In optometry, precision and attention to detail are vital, making honing the skill of history-taking especially crucial. This Study Guide takes a unique approach by presenting a variety of fictional characters, each with their own thoughtfully crafted case history. These characters serve as valuable tools for educators and learners, offering a dynamic platform to practice and refine the art of gathering comprehensive patient information.

For Lecturers:
As a lecturer, you play a key role in shaping the future healthcare workforce. This Study Guide equips you with a diverse array of fictional patients, each with detailed case histories. Whether you teach optometry, medicine, or a related discipline, integrate these characters into your curriculum. Use them as exam cases to challenge your students' diagnostic abilities and foster critical thinking. The scenarios cover a range of ocular conditions, preparing your students for the complexities they may face in their careers.

For Students:
Entering the healthcare field requires not just theory but practical skills. This Study Guide serves as your interactive guide to mastering the art of history-taking. Each fictional character presents a puzzle for you to solve, providing an opportunity to apply your knowledge in a simulated clinical setting. Practice these cases individually or with peers to enhance communication skills, develop a systematic approach to history-taking, and gain confidence in diagnostic abilities.

A Resource for All:
Whether you're a seasoned pro or an eager learner, "*History & Symptoms: The Eye Examination*" is crafted to be accessible. The characters span a diverse range of ages, backgrounds, and eye conditions, ensuring relevance in various healthcare contexts. The cases are designed to be engaging and relatable, making the learning process both educational and enjoyable.

Cases were crafted not only to help train for the taking of a case history, but to incorporate real components found within histories that correspond to the presenting condition. This is in the hope that students will identify patterns and common answers in certain presentations, enabling them to feel primed when facing real patients in pre-registration and beyond.

Whilst all cases, names and patients featured within this book are fictional, the fictional characters within are based on real-life presentations and personality types that exist in primary care optometry.

Why is taking a case history important?

In the world of eye care, chatting with a patient about their history and symptoms is like unlocking a treasure trove of information that will help you in your appointment. It's a crucial part of the job because it helps us understand why the patient is here, and what's bothering them the most, and can even give us clues about what might be going on with their eyes.

When a patient walks into the optometrist's office, the first thing we want to know is, "*Why are they here?*" That's where their history comes in handy. Unlike other doctors, who might deal with obvious symptoms, eye issues can be a bit sneakier. The patient might be struggling with blurry vision, discomfort, or maybe even headaches, each with a handful of potential causes. Getting to the bottom of why they've come in helps us focus on what to check during their eye exam.

Knowing the patient's main concerns is just as important. Sometimes, they might come in for one thing but have other worries they didn't mention right away. For example, someone complaining about occasional blurriness might also be dealing with flashes of light or other unusual visual complaints. The more we know, the better we can figure out what's going on.

But the best bit of taking a good history means that the patient can tell us a lot based on what they're feeling and experiencing. Their symptoms, or how they describe what's happening, give us a heads-up on what might be up with their eyes. Someone with sudden, intense eye pain, along with a headache and nausea, is dealing with a different situation than someone slowly feeling their eyes getting dry and irritated. Listening to these details not only helps spot the main problem but also gives us clues about other possible issues.

Therefore, it is unsurprising that a good case history can sometimes lead us to tentatively diagnose the patient well before we dive into the formal eye tests. By putting together what the patient says, their symptoms, and our experience, we can start to paint a picture of what's happening. For example, if someone talks about a slow reduction in the quality of their vision, trouble seeing at night, and experiencing glare, it might suggest a cataract. Essentially, it provides us a heads-up on what we can expect to find once we start testing.

But, here's the catch – if we don't ask the right questions or if we miss some details, we might get the wrong idea. A poor history might mean we overlook something important, misinterpret something the patient has said and ultimately jump to the wrong conclusion.

And there's something else to watch out for – red herrings. These are distractions that can throw us off course. A patient might mention something that seems important but is not connected to their main eye issue. A good case history, involving a good mix of open and probing questions, helps us sort through these distractions and stay focused on what truly matters to the patient.

In a nutshell, when we chat with patients about their eye history and symptoms, it's more than just going through the motions of an eye appointment. It's having a friendly conversation that helps us understand why they've come, what's bothering them, and what their symptoms mean. Their story guides us to possible diagnoses and helps us avoid mistakes. As optometrists, we should value these chats because they're the key to giving great eye care!

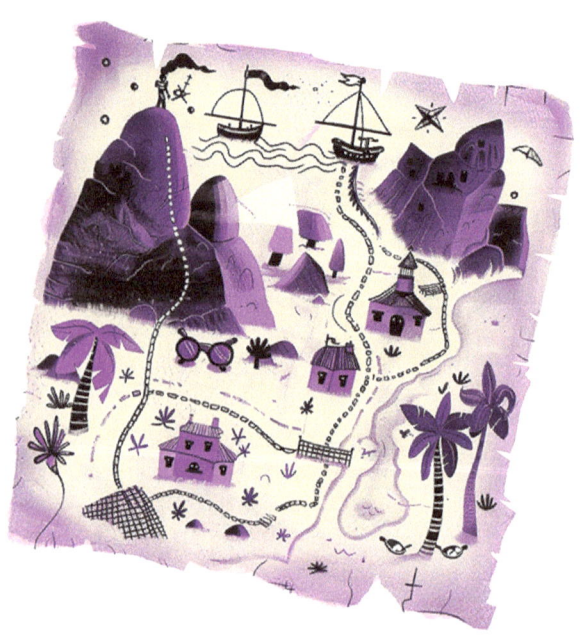

How to effectively take a case history

In this chapter of the book, we lift the bonnet on the art of taking a case history, without delving too deeply into the optometric side of things. The ability to take a case history cannot be switched on without experience and practice; it can take many encounters, situations, and reflections to be fully confident in asking the right things in the right way to best extract the information that you need to effectively conduct an eye examination. This is why university courses, The College of Optometrists, The General Optical Council, and all other optical organisations that have educational input emphasise communication and case histories as important learning objectives. This chapter is a brief guide on factors that can boost your ability to take case histories.

The SOLER Model

The SOLER model (Egan, 1975) is a key set of rules for communicating with your patient during a case history, as they enable you to show that you are paying attention to them and are invested in what they have to say.

SOLER is an acronym and the letters stand for:

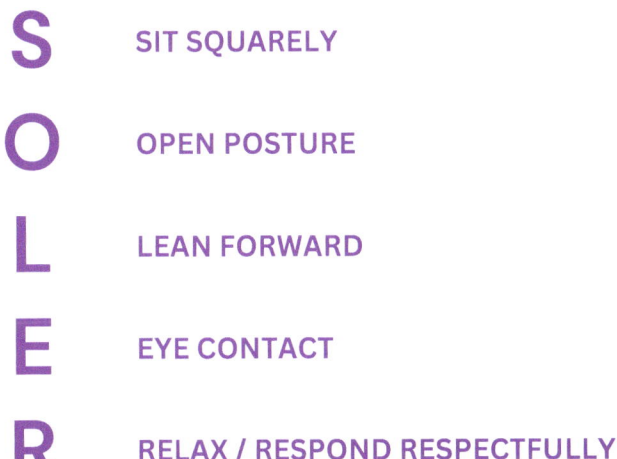

S   SIT SQUARELY

O   OPEN POSTURE

L   LEAN FORWARD

E   EYE CONTACT

R   RELAX / RESPOND RESPECTFULLY

We will now look at the SOLER model in a little more detail:

S

Sit Squarely
When interacting with a patient, position yourself at the same level as them. Avoid appearing dominant or intimidating. Sit squarely, maintaining an open and attentive posture.

O

Open Posture
Keep your body language "open." Avoid crossing your arms or legs, as this can signal defensiveness or conflict. An open posture fosters a welcoming environment.

L

Lean Forward
Leaning toward the patient demonstrates interest and engagement. It conveys that you're genuinely listening. However, be cautious not to invade their personal space.

E

Eye Contact
Maintain appropriate eye contact. It shows attentiveness without being overly intense. Remember that cultural norms influence eye contact interpretation and as such be aware of what is considered too little and too much at any given encounter.

R

Relax
Display relaxation in your demeanor. It communicates that you have time for the patient and aren't rushed. Confidence and respect emanate from a relaxed stance.

In some models, the R can represent "Respond Respectfully", which means just that. Be courteous, respectful and mindful of your patients' culture and wishes.

The SOLER model provides a great starting point for those wishing to improve their communication skills, but should not be used alone when you are planning to interact with patients. The following pages will look at other techniques you can utilise to effectively communicate with your patients.

Active Listening

We listen to things every day. Listening is simply being aware or focused on a sound that our ears have picked up. Whilst this natural skill can be performed motionless and with our eyes closed, to an onlooker, someone doing this may not appear as if they are listening or perhaps be asleep. Likewise, if you are at a doctor's appointment and they are typing away at their computer or looking through previous notes, they may very well be listening, however, your perception of them may be that they are distracted or not paying attention to what you are saying.

This is where active listening comes in. Active listening can be likened to listening, but instead of just being a passive skill, it brings you into the conversation and allows you to engage with the person you are talking with. The engagement will need to come from many levels, but the person you are engaging with will understand that you are listening to them, aiding in the development of empathy and care.

To demonstrate active listening, you must:

Provide your full attention
This involves participating in the conversation and showing genuine interest in what they say and do. It also involves avoiding distractions, so ensure you aren't using your phone/tablet, try to minimise checking back through case notes, and make sure you look at your patients and be square to them when talking with them.

Give non-verbal clues
As you may have heard repeatedly, a significant amount of what we are communicating doesn't come from what we say, but from our body language. Show you are listening to your patients by nodding, keeping eye contact, and facing them appropriately. These clues convey to your patient that they are being listened to and understood.

Avoid interruptions

Interruptions can disrupt the flow of your conversation and create distractions. This may lead to important information not being heard or even misheard. Try not to have anything in the room that can interrupt the appointment (so make sure your mobile phone is away!)

Additionally, try not to interrupt the patient when they are talking to you. If you speak over or interject too frequently, you will be seen as hurrying the patient or not caring about what they have to say. This can cause a reduction in rapport and can lead to difficulties later on in the appointment.

Paraphrase

It is useful to paraphrase what your patient has just told you. This not only helps make what they have told you clear in your head but also demonstrates to the patient that you have listened and understood appropriately. This also provides them a chance to correct you if they think that you haven't understood them.

Empathy

Put yourself in your patient's shoes. How would you feel if you were the one talking to you? Are they anxious to be here? Are they upset by something? Taking the time to put empathy into your conversation and actively adapting to your patients' needs will demonstrate to them that you genuinely care and are there to help them.

Clarification

Don't be afraid to ask further questions if the patient says something that you don't understand or may require further information about. Asking these extra probing questions shows that you have understood what has been said so far, or you may need to have further information to understand what has been said better. This shows that you're paying attention. However, repeatedly asking for clarification or reiterating points that have been previously made could suggest that you're not fully engaged.

In addition to active listening, structuring your questions appropriately can help boost your efficiency of extracting the most information from your patient in the shortest amount of time.

Start With Open Questions

Open questions are important because they create a welcoming and inclusive environment for effective communication. Unlike close-ended questions that prompt simple yes or no answers, open-ended questions encourage detailed and expressive responses. This is valuable in various contexts, including healthcare, as it allows for a more comprehensive understanding of the individual's thoughts, feelings, and experiences.

By using open-ended questions, you invite your patient to share their perspective without constraints. This not only promotes a deeper level of engagement but also fosters trust and a sense of collaboration. It's akin to opening a door to a rich and nuanced conversation where people feel heard and understood. In healthcare settings, like optometry, this approach is particularly crucial as it helps uncover subtle symptoms, emotions, and details that might be missed with closed questioning. Ultimately, open questions enhance the quality of communication, paving the way for more accurate diagnoses and personalised care.

Follow With Closed Questions

Follow-up closed questions play a crucial role in communication by delving deeper into specific details. Instead of stopping at the surface, these questions aim to uncover more about the individual's experiences. For instance, asking "When did you first notice these symptoms?" or "Have you experienced any changes in your vision recently?" acts like a magnifying glass, zooming in on the timeline and specifics.

These probing questions help in pinpointing important information, offering a more detailed snapshot of the situation. It's akin to turning the dial to focus the lens, ensuring that no crucial details are overlooked. In healthcare, such probing questions are instrumental, allowing for a more precise understanding of symptoms and contributing to a thorough and accurate assessment.

Prioritise Your Questions!

It may seem obvious but prioritise your patients' questions based on their chief complaints and reasons for visit. If you have a patient presenting with red flags that are likely to require an emergency referral, you want the most information about that chief complaint and will want to structure your history and appointment around that. You will waste valuable time and appear less empathetic if you are asking about the amount of time they are on the computer or determining if it was their aunt or uncle who had a cataract when the patient has symptoms suggestive of a retinal detachment or foreign body.

This also applies to routine appointments. If they present with issues with their distance vision, but everything else appears fine, then adapt your questions around finding out why their distance vision isn't as good (but ensure you do perform a complete history covering key aspects of an eye examination).

Maintain a Structured Approach

A structured case history is one where very little ends up being left out. Knowing what questions to ask and when to ask them sets a good foundation for obtaining the most relevant information for the appointment. You will find that some parts of the case history just flow into one another, allowing for a conversational feel and removing the staccato of endless questioning.

The structure also will aid in building your patter, that is, the "muscle memory" that comes with doing a task frequently. Having a good patter develop over time will mean you know what to say, and how to word it to get the most information from each question and you'll never be left wondering what to ask next.

A well-structured history adds ease to the record-keeping requirements as well. If you record things in a set way, if you need to refer to a point made during the eye exam (or at a later date), you will be able to quickly identify where the relevant points are in your records. Furthermore, having this set layout will aid you in being conversational, as any relevant points raised in different parts of the history can be recorded in their relevant spot, allowing for less questioning and more demonstration of active listening as you won't ask for information that the patient has already provided.

Social Sensitivity

Social sensitivity is a vital aspect of communication, urging us to recognise and respect diverse backgrounds. It involves being attuned to cultural differences and adjusting our approach accordingly. This means acknowledging various perspectives and communication styles and creating an inclusive space where everyone feels understood. In healthcare, including optometry, cultural sensitivity extends beyond ethnicity, encompassing other protected groups such as those with disabilities or different gender identities.

It is recognising that individuals from different backgrounds may have unique needs and preferences. Adapting our approach ensures that our interactions are not only respectful but also tailored to each person, fostering an environment where everyone, regardless of cultural or personal distinctions, receives the care and attention they deserve.

Some key points to consider include:

- Use appropriate language and terminology.
- Sit appropriately and avoid "manspreading*".
- Allowing the use of translators or allowing extra time where communication barriers exist.
- Avoid assuming, such as "You are W therefore you must follow Y and therefore I must do Z".
- Be respectful and avoid allowing personal opinions or prejudices to come into the appointment.
- Ask for personal preferences where appropriate (e.g. pronouns).
- Be mindful of religious holidays and faiths when managing patients and their treatment plans.

---

*Manspreading occurs when a man sits with his legs wide apart, occupying more space than usual. It's recommended to avoid this posture, as it can come across as impolite and may even seem intimidating to your patient.

Be Adaptable

This follows directly from social sensitivity. Every patient you see will be unique and often you will need to adapt your personality and style to best address the person in front of you.

Some patients may have hearing difficulties, so you may need to speak louder and clearer than you normally do. Some may be from a different area of the country and find your accent hard to understand, so you may have to work at suppressing your normal way of speaking. Some patients may be shy or anxious and not appreciate your domineering questioning (so tone it back and show empathy) and likewise, some patients have very extroverted or aggressive personalities that may require you to up your energy to match them.

Being able to recognise the patient in front of you and to adapt to their needs is a skill that does take time to develop, but mastering this ability will increase the efficiency of your tests and allow for rapport to build rapidly.

Summarise

Being able to summarise what your patient has told you is a critical skill in both demonstrating active listening and for clarifying to yourself what this patient will require from you during the appointment. Periodically summarising to your patient will help to identify what the patient is here for and allow them to add further information (or correct you) if required.

Effective Time Management

Applying the aforementioned strategies will greatly enhance your time management skills. While I've added some extra tips that could further refine your time allocation, keep in mind that some may be better suited for experienced practitioners in a primary care clinic rather than those still learning the skill of history taking in an academic environment.

Use templates
A template for a case history can be used to help prompt you to cover key aspects of the history. These may be templates on paper records or on electronic record systems.

Practice and training
The more cases you take, the better you become at taking them. Whilst learning be sure to hone this skill throughout your course and don't fall into the trap of thinking the other clinical skills that are taught have more importance. Remember, you can usually tentatively diagnose a patient through a thorough case history in most cases!

Staff support
Ask staff to indicate the reason for the visit on the diary, allowing you to prepare for what the chief complaint may be ahead of calling them into the room. This can help mentally prepare for any adaptations you may need going forward. Additionally, ask your reception staff to annotate the booking with any significant information that will aid your appointment.

Work "set clinics" (e.g. contact lens clinic, eye exam clinic, emergency clinics)
These set clinic types will help you manage your workload effectively as you will keep in the mindset of the type of optometric service that you are trying to offer. It will also prevent you from muddling your questions during history and symptoms (such as asking contact lens specific questions to those who don't have contact lenses). Whilst these set clinics are often seen in the multiples, in some situations this may not be possible due to the nature of how that particular practice works.

Pre-appointment forms
Some practices may send pre-appointment forms to the patient prior to the appointment where patients can add their key information regarding the case history. If this is the case, you may even save time on taking the history as the majority of the information will be there. That said, you MUST review, record and confirm this history with the patient, which may take longer than performing your case history from scratch.

Utilise previous records
If the patient is an existing patient to the practice, you should have access to their previous record cards - so read through them in advance. These previous records will provide you with a heads up on what to expect in this appointment - especially if your patient is in earlier than the expected recall date.

Many details in a case history will remain constant (e.g. a patient having a heart attack in 2012 won't suddenly not have had a heart attack in 2012!) so keep this in mind when asking questions.

Finally, avoid using "as before" on a new record. Things do change often and if you do refer back, having 10 pages of "as before" may make it tricky to locate the information and may not be reliable. It may also look like you haven't actually asked the questions.

What to include on a primary care case history?

When a patient walks through the doors of a primary care optometry practice, their story begins to unfold, and it's our job to listen carefully. A well-crafted case history not only guides the examination process but also helps us understand the individual beyond their eyes. Let's explore the key elements that should be part of a thorough case history.

Please note, this Study Guide looks primarily at patients attending an eye examination. In time, I plan to expand this to be a series on patients presenting for various appointments, including contact lenses and low vision appointments.

Reason for Visit
Start at the beginning – why did the patient decide to come in? Are they experiencing specific issues like blurry vision, discomfort, or changes in their eyesight? Are they merely just answering your recall letter and having no specific issues at all?

Knowing why your patient has attended gives you a focus for the eye examination. Think of it as them setting you a problem or a task for you to solve and make sure you solve and address this at the end of the appointment.

The term "Reason for Visit" is often denoted by the acronym "RFV" on a record card, but can also be denoted by "CC" meaning "chief complaint". Ideally you should have both of these documented as they will present for an appointment for one thing, but one particular symptom may be most pressing.

Last Eye Examination
Knowing when the patient had their last eye check is crucial. It provides insight into their eye health history and helps track changes over time. Additionally, if a patient is in sooner than their expected recall date, there is often a problem than needs addressing.

Furthermore, in cases such as NHS eligibility or health insurance-funded appointments, patients may only be eligible to claim an eye examination routinely at a set interval. Seeing them earlier may warrant them to self-fund or require us to further assess their eligibility to be seen earlier than expected.

On a record card, you may see the acronym "LEE", which stands for "last eye examination".

Subjective Assessment of Vision
Ask how the patient finds their vision. How do they feel about their distance vision? Near vision? Is anything bothering them in between? Knowing if there is a problem with any of these distances could give valuable insight into what they may be struggling with and provide hints to any changes that you may find in refraction.

An example of this is someone aged 45 complaining that they cannot see up close, hinting that they are becoming presbyopic and require a near prescription, or a child struggling to see the whiteboard at school, meaning they are likely to require a myopic correction.

On my records, I usually write "DV", "IV" and "NV" that stands for "distance vision", "intermediate vision" and "near vision" respectively. Next to each of these I note down how they find vision at these distances. It provides me a quick reference point when summarising the eye test and explaining my findings as I can pin-point a cause to their subjective findings.

Red Flag Symptoms

Certain symptoms are a clear cause to investigate further to rule out more serious issues that may require management and/or referral. The red flag questions you should ask about are:

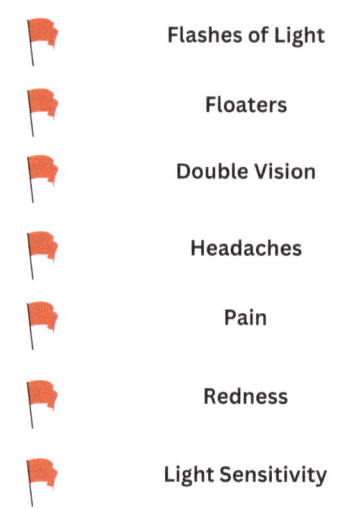

- Flashes of Light
- Floaters
- Double Vision
- Headaches
- Pain
- Redness
- Light Sensitivity

As these symptoms can have significant underlying causes, asking about these and recording if they have or haven't experienced these symptoms will aid your examination and help protect you should a problem occur later and you need to evidence that these symptoms were not present at the examination.

If any of these symptoms are present (or there are any symptoms present at all), you should follow up the symptoms with the "LOFTSEA" questions (discussed overleaf) to further understand the symptoms and to allow you to investigate their origins further.

LOFTSEA

You may be wondering what the word "LOFTSEA" is, but it is in fact an acronym to help remind you of the follow up questions you need to ask in response to symptoms. All symptoms reported should be investigated via this acronym to fully understand the way the symptoms are affecting your patient.

L **LOCATION** — Where does the symptom take place? The right eye, the left eye or both? On the conjunctiva or on the eyelid? Knowing where the symptom occurs lets you know where to investigate.

O **ONSET** — When did the symptom start happening? Was it today, last week or did it start years ago? A more recent onset usually will mean something has changed and needs more urgent attention, but don't neglect historic or chronic symptoms.

F **FREQUENCY** — How often do the symptoms occur? Symptoms of a high frequency are more likely to be concerning to the patient, or more likely to have an active cause, but do remember to investigate occasional and rarely experienced symptoms too!

T **TYPE** — Ask them to describe the symptoms more. Is it double or is it blurry? If double, describe if the two images are side by side or on top of one another? If they are reporting discomfort, is it a mild niggle or is it extremely painful?

S **SELF-TREATMENT** — What measures has the patient taken to alleviate the symptoms? If their vision is blurry far away without glasses, have they tried their distance glasses and has that worked? Do dry eye drops help their dry eye? Do painkillers help with their headaches?

E **EFFECT ON LIFE** — Ask how their symptoms are affecting their life? Is that headache just a niggle they can work through, or do they need time off work? Is the light-sensitivity so bad they cannot go outside? You can use this to help form a management plan.

A **ASSOCIATED SYMPTOMS** — Do the symptoms occur by themselves, or do other symptoms occur with them? The more symptoms that a patient reports at this stage provides more pieces of the puzzle that you can piece together in order to form a tentative diagnosis.

Ocular History
Ask and understand the patient's eye history. Have they ever visited the ophthalmology department or eye hospital? Have they ever had a diagnosis of eye disease? I recommend specifically asking about glaucoma as a diagnosis as it opens the door to further questioning about their glaucoma status and identification of further risk factors for the disease if they do not currently have glaucoma.

The ocular history will aid in your assessment and may even throw you some potential causes for their reason for visit. A patient that presents with a red and painful eye that has a history of cataract surgery 2 weeks ago may point towards a complication of the surgery. Similarly, if they say they are aware of cataracts forming from the previous eye examination, that slow and gradual clouding of their vision may be attributed to this.

It can also help rule out significant problems with the eye. Take a patient with dense amblyopia with a historic best corrected acuity of 6/60. Knowing this at the start of the appointment will prevent panic or concern when you are refracting the patient and they cannot get better than the 6/60 line.

Furthermore, knowing if they are treating their eyes with any medication can help you decide if the management of the condition is appropriate. Someone saying they have symptoms of dry eye and they haven't been advised to treat it may benefit from that suggestion when you conclude the appointment.

Ocular history is noted as "OH" or "POH" on the record card.

Family Ocular History
Family matters. Ask about eye conditions in their close relatives. Some eye conditions have genetic components that may increase the risk of your patient developing the same condition. In some cases, such as a family history of glaucoma, you may wish to run additional tests to ensure glaucoma isn't present. Furthermore, some contracts may require you to perform these additional tests on at-risk patients for you to claim the fee for the appointment.

Asking about family history can give insight into your patients' and raise an opportunity to discuss modifiable risk factors with them (such as stopping smoking if they have a family history of macular degeneration). Additionally, it provides educational moments to ensure your patient is aware to discuss their ocular health with their family.

I **STRONGLY** advise asking about glaucoma and macular degeneration in the family as these two conditions are common and, if present in the family, would warrant you performing the additional tests to rule them out. If there is no history of any eye disease, ensure you write this negative finding on the record card.

Family ocular history is usually noted as "FOH" on the record card.

General Health

You must also ask questions regarding their general health. Patients might wonder how questions regarding their overall health relate to their eye condition. It's important to explain that systemic diseases like diabetes, hypertension, and high cholesterol can increase the risk of developing eye-related issues. Additionally, some of the medication used to treat their general health complaints can cause ocular side effects. Therefore it is imperative to cover this section of the case history in detail.

In general, it is advisable to ask openly to ensure that any significant health condition has a chance to be mentioned, but ideally, you would like to make note if the patient is diabetic, hypertensive or has any heart conditions (and it is worth asking about these conditions directly if they say "all is fine"). As these conditions can have significant implications on the eyes noting a positive or negative finding is key.

If the patient is diabetic, be sure to ask what type, how long they have been diabetic for and how the control of their blood sugars is. These answers can significantly alter their risk factors for diabetic retinopathy. You will also need to ask whether they are being seen annually by the diabetic retinal screening teams, as this could affect your management and recall for the patient.

Furthermore, being aware of the symptoms of major health issues can help ensure your patients get the help they need. Brain tumours, thyroid problems, liver failure, and cancer are all things that have been picked up in my clinics from discussion in case history and prompt referral to their primary care provider has ensured the relevant tests and diagnoses have been identified.

In this post-covid world, GP appointments can be difficult to obtain, and many patients may simply not attempt to get an appointment to urgently assess concerning symptoms. You may be the first healthcare professional that you see and, as such, picking up on something that doesn't seem right and referring them to their GP could just save their life. Our care does not just stop at the eyes!

General health is often denoted as "GH" on the record card.

Allergies

Allergies are an area I often see neglected on a record card. It is a vital question to ask as allergies can cause life-threatening consequences if not identified appropriately.

We will use certain drugs and dyes on patients in the diagnostic process and, should we use one and the patient has a known allergy to it, you may well find yourself in a legal mess! ALWAYS find out about your patients' allergies and document that you have asked.

Furthermore, if you do have to refer your patient knowing that a patient has a specific allergy will aid their journey through ophthalmology, where they are more likely to encounter the allergen than in your testing room (i.e. more exposure to medications, latex and hospital food!)

Medications
Asking about medication is an important component of any case history. There are several reasons as to why it is vital to ask about the medication that your patient is taking:

Ocular side effects: Being able to understand the common (and some uncommon) side effects of systemic medication can aid in your examination should your patient present with certain symptoms or may explain the presence of certain signs that you may see during your assessment.

Systemic side effects: Whilst you will be mainly focused on ocular health, some medications can cause significant side effects for the patient. Being aware of what your patient is stating during the history and knowing the medication they are taking could mean that you are the person that identifies the issues with a certain medication, which you can then refer to the prescriber for consideration and action (an example of this could be a patient with significant headaches caused by codeine withdrawal symptoms from unintentional addiction).

Knowing the treatment and management that you may be able to implement. If you are a therapeutic optometrist, you may prescribe medications such as antibiotics or steroids. These medications may interact with medications that your patient may be taking and as such care would need to be taken to ensure you don't bring the patient to harm when prescribing the medication used to treat the eye problem (e.g. modified dosage or alternative medication may be required).

To fill in gaps in the patient's general health history. There will be times when you will see patients that tell you that their general health is fine and that they are healthy. They may then produce a list of the medication that they are taking, and on the list, you see medication that is used to treat diabetes, hypertension, and heart issues. This can then prompt you to ask specifically about these issues to ensure the case history is complete.

Family General Health
Family general health is a piece of the puzzle too – in a similar way that family ocular health can provide information regarding the health of your patient. For example, if most of the patient's family got diagnosed with diabetes in their 50s and the patient is in their sixties with the odd dot or blot haemorrhage, you would likely be considering the cause to be diabetic in nature.

Understanding the health of a family member with ocular diseases can shed light on the reasons behind their eye condition. For example, consider a patient whose mother has wet macular degeneration. However, the mother was also hypertensive, smoked 40 cigarettes a day, and had numerous basal cell carcinomas due to UV damage. In such cases, health and lifestyle factors often play a more significant role in macular degeneration risk than purely genetic causes. It's essential not to assume this correlation, but investigating thoroughly and ruling out disease indicators can help reassure patients who worry excessively about their risk of AMD.

Family General Health is often denoted as "FGH" on the record card.

Occupation
The occupation is a point that many people tend to forget to ask but it does form an important part of the case history. If you consider the visual demands for a variety of jobs, are they all the same or do they differ? Would the visual demands of an electrician be the same as that a commercial pilot or a hair stylist?

Taking the time to ask your patients about their occupation and occupational needs will ensure the tests you perform are at the required distances and angles, with the ability to advise and prescribe accordingly to maximise your patients' vision at work and provide them with clear and comfortable vision.

You should also be aware of the visual standards for these roles. Some roles, such as a heavy goods vehicle driver will need to have a higher standard acuity to drive their HGV than a car and as such being aware of what your patient does for a living can put you in a better position to advise them of the implications of changes to their vision means to them and their roles.

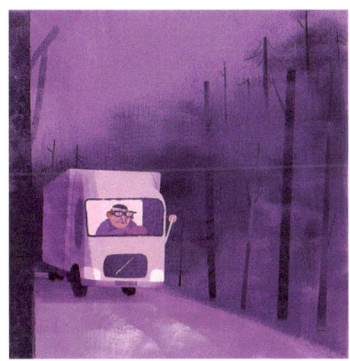

Hobbies

All occupations all have their own specific needs, and the same goes for hobbies, interests and leisure activities too! The visual demands of a chess player will be different to that of an artist, video gamer or astronomer. Understanding the needs of your patient will help you prescribe and advise accordingly, allowing you to also hand over to the dispensing team additional information on how to correct any visual concerns.

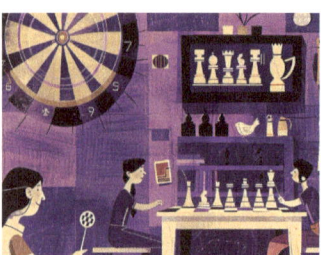

In my experience, discussing hobbies is an effective way to connect with patients. By sharing personal experiences and asking about unique or unusual hobbies, you demonstrate genuine interest in them as individuals, rather than just someone conducting eye tests for payment.

You will also understand that your patients are individuals and, on occasion, provide insight into hobbies, charities, events and services that you wouldn't have even thought about searching for.

Visual Display Unit (VDU) Usage

The modern world is dominated by screens. If we aren't using one to work from, we are using them to catch up with the latest shows, or messaging friends on our phones. Screen usage requires good near focus and if your patient is on the VDU for a significant amount of time, they may start having eyestrain or have issues keeping near focus.

Our blink rate also deteriorates when we are using a screen, meaning that we often find ourselves staring. This in turn can impact tear quality over the ocular surface, leading to dry eye and eye irritation. Having knowledge of VDU usage will aid in your investigation into symptoms that may indicate dry eye, allowing you to formulate this into any management strategies.

VDU usage can also provide an understanding to symptoms of blurring in pre-presbyopic patients, as increased near demands can cause overload of their accommodative system, leading to accommodative spasm and other binocular vision-related symptoms.

Whilst it seems a small question with little meaning, knowing the number of hours your patient is behind a screen can be the key to unlocking the cause of their symptoms.

Social and Lifestyle
Asking questions about their social life can also be key to identifying any issues your patient may be having. This can feature as part of the "hobbies" section, but identifying if your patient smokes or drinks alcohol can be useful insight. Smoking increases the risk of eye diseases and can accelerate the development of cataracts, whilst drinking can cause an imbalance in overall health and lead to other ocular issues.

With the guidance to encourage people to better look after themselves due to overstretched and under-resourced health services, using this moment of rapport building to encourage patients to consider their lifestyle choices and nudge them to stop smoking or reduce alcohol consumption can go a long way towards increasing the long-term well-being of your patients.

Driving
Driving is an important aspect of most of your patients' lives. Whether they drive locally, commute, use it to transport their family or even work as a professional driver, good vision is required to ensure they are not risking themselves or others when they get behind the wheel.

Furthermore, it is important to understand that there are strict driving standards for vision. These vary from country to country and between classes of vehicle (you will be pleased to know that the vision requirements for HGV and passenger buses are MUCH more stringent than that required for a car).

Knowing if your patient is driving, what they are driving and if they have visual correction to meet those requirements is vital to ensure you are advising them correctly and, should the findings of your test indicate otherwise, have the discussions around their visual ability to meet the required standards.

I always ensure I document any discussion around driving - including if they wear any form of correction when they drive. This will not only ensure you provide the correct guidance to them, but it will also help serve as a discussion point when deciding if you need to recommend an update to their current optical prescription.

Contact Lens Use
Whilst contact lenses are not directly involved in a standard eye examination, understanding your patient's history with them will aid in diagnosing any potential symptomatic eye and visual problems that arise. It will also provide an opportunity to tackle any non-compliance to contact lens use and, should the patient not already use contact lenses, it opens up a conversation about fitting them as part of their management.

It is easy to forget, but try and ask about contact lenses at every appropriate appointment!

Summary
Integrating these elements, a comprehensive case history becomes a roadmap. Each detail contributes to the patient's narrative, guiding you, as the optometrist, in understanding not only their current eye health but also the broader context of their life. This transforms the routine eye examination into a personalised experience, where the patient's unique story unfolds, ensuring thorough consideration of every aspect of their eye health.

By actively listening to patients' stories and exploring various dimensions, primary care optometry adopts a holistic approach that goes far beyond just examination of their eyes. It delves into the individual behind the eyes, fostering a more personalised and effective approach to health and eye care.

Case Study Scripts

The main body of this book will focus on providing you the opportunity to take case histories, with a wide selection of fictional patients with unique personalities and backgrounds.

Whilst designed to be a practical study tool, where you can work with a colleague or peer, the case scenarios can also be read as a transcript to help mentally cement the flow of a case history and understand the structure within. Following each script is a reflection on some of the key points of the case history, which will help develop your critical evaluation skills.

Please read the following to ensure you get the best out of these case scenarios. Each one has been carefully selected to cover a range of presentations, personality types and underlying pathology to expose you to how patients will present to you in primary care.

How to use these case scenarios

Advice for the student/person acting as practitioner
This guide is designed for practical study and as a useful starting point for practising case histories with fictional characters, especially if you're gearing up for an exam featuring the taking of a case history.

You will act as an optometrist, taking a history from a colleague/peer/friend or relative, who will use the transcript as a guide for answering your questions. Please treat this as a real life scenario, recording your findings, treating your partner respectfully and acting professionally. You may need to adapt how you take the case history in response to the patient's personality.

After the session, take a moment to compare your notes with the provided case history. Assess how well you covered the necessary categories and information you have gleaned from the conversation.

When you're feeling confident, try timing yourself – aim for your case history to be completed within 5 minutes, as often you will not have longer than this in your clinic. The 5 minute-mark is also the typical length of time that you have in an OSCE or SOPE setting. This skill-building exercise helps streamline your approach, leaving more time to focus on understanding and addressing your patients' needs.

If your partner can, they may choose to use the case histories of a given patient but try to act in different ways to how the cases have been portrayed (e.g. making an aggressive case more mellow, or vice versa). This will provide you with further experience in this vital practical skill.

Advice for the actor/ person portraying the patient
Most of the key information required for you to fulfil your role is given, but there may be times where the practitioner will ask a question that may not have a given answer. If it isn't written down, it is ok to say "I don't know" or to say "no" to any question asked. This is because in real life, patients frequently aren't aware of some of their case history and as such, having these moments will help the practitioner understand that there isn't always an answer to their question and will force them to utilise their problem-solving skills to work with the information that they do have available.

It can also be tricky memorising the script if you are doing a number of these case scenarios, especially when revising. As such, if there are any moments that you need to check the script for accuracy, do so! Patients will often search for prescriptions, old pairs of glasses or their latest hospital letter during the history-taking – so this could be likened to these moments. Whilst this could be slightly frustrating for the practitioner, it is very much a reflection of what happens in an appointment.

Do not fear giving a wrong answer. Patients sometimes get their history wrong. Let the practitioner probe if there are parts of the history that do not add up. Do your best to stick to the script, but don't worry if you make a mistake!

Finally, be observant of the person taking the history from you. Are they being too aggressive with their questioning or holding back on asking some of the more probing questions. Feed back to them at the end of every scenario as this will help them grow.

Advice to observers
Studying is not always done alone or in pairs and, should you wish to use these scenarios in group revision, please do!

Whilst it is primarily a two-person activity, don't be afraid to work in groups of three or four, where anyone not directly involved in the scenario can observe, take notes and reflect on the activity at hand.

Take notes of what the practitioner is doing in response. Maybe they are being too quick in their questioning, or too quiet, or not asking enough. Making notes and feeding this back will aid their development and help improve their confidence in this skill.

You may also wish to practice recording what is being answered. Whilst you may not be asking the questions, you can benefit from the skill of taking notes and familiarising yourself with what and how to record patient responses.

Finally, you can reflect on what you have observed and what you would do differently. Watching people perform the skill you are honing can be great experience, so please do utilise this resource in this way!

For those studying alone

This book primarily serves as a practical tool, but the reflections following each case offer valuable insights. These reflections dissect various aspects of the case history, shedding light on their significance in real-world practice.

While no single case history can comprehensively cover every area of interest, the goal across this book is to delve into why specific parts of the case history matter and provides additional insights as to why you need to ask a range of questions covering a wide range of topics.

Consider these reflections as nuggets of wisdom drawn from the complexities of clinical encounters. They will enrich your understanding, shaping you into a more astute and compassionate practitioner.

Advice for Lecturers, Teachers, Assessors and Supervisors

Feel free to incorporate these scripts and case scenarios into your lesson planning and practical sessions. As educators, you can leverage these resources to enhance your teaching and assessment methods. Here's how:

1. **Lesson Planning:**
   - Integrate these case scenarios into your lectures or workshops.
   - Use them as teaching aids to illustrate real-world situations.
   - Encourage active discussion and problem-solving among students.
2. **Assessment Tools:**
   - Utilise these cases within exam stations, written exam papers, or other assessments.
   - Ensure that students apply their knowledge and critical thinking skills.
   - Assess their ability to analyse and respond to clinical scenarios.
3. **Supervision and Case History Taking:**
   - If you supervise undergraduate clinics or pre-registration settings, these scripts can be valuable tools.
   - Guide students in understanding the importance of specific questions during patient assessments.
   - Use the scenarios to evaluate their proficiency in gathering relevant case history information.

- **Licensing Considerations:**
   - Remember that your purchase of this book grants you the right to use these cases within your educational institution.
   - However, refrain from using them for commercial purposes or selling them externally.
   - The focus should remain on teaching and learning within your specific establishment.

Remember, these resources are designed to enhance the learning experience and foster clinical competence.

Case Study Selection 1

Routine Presentations

In this section, we explore routine eye tests—a fundamental aspect of optometry. These scenarios mirror everyday practice, where patients provide minimal case history but may exhibit minor symptoms requiring further investigation. From common issues like blepharitis and meibomian gland dysfunction to early cataracts, these cases form the core of your optometric encounters.

As you review these straightforward case histories, you'll recognise the importance of efficient patient management. Addressing mild headaches and eyestrain becomes crucial, highlighting optometry's role in overall eye and systemic health.

This section underscores the significance of mastering history-taking during routine eye tests. Discerning subtle patient-reported symptoms is essential for comprehensive care. Even seemingly routine examinations demand a keen eye, a systematic approach, and a commitment to meticulous patient well-being.

Please remember that all of the following cases are fictional patients, but representing real-world presentations. Any similarities to people, real or fictional, is purely co-incidental.

Case #001: David

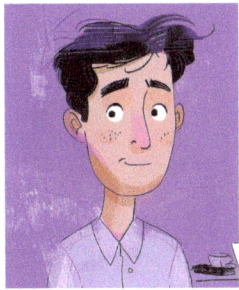

Composition – For the person acting as this patient:

David is a friendly, easy-going and relaxed 32-year-old IT consultant. He is helpful and pleased to be fitted in for an eye examination today. David provides information easily and answers are generally free-flowing upon questioning.

The blue text provides an example of the type of response you should provide to this question

Reason for Visit	"I'm here because you sent me a letter to say I am due an eye examination"
Last Eye Examination	"2 years ago - here"
Subjective Visual Assessment	"I'm not noticing any problems, distance, near and intermediate vision is fine. I don't need any glasses to help me see"
Key Symptoms	"No symptoms for me!" (No to any red flag symptoms asked about)
LOFTSEA	N/A (as no symptoms to investigate)
Ocular History	"None - I've never worn glasses, no injuries, no eye diseases, no hospital visits. No eye issues at all."
Family Ocular History	"There are no significant eye problems. My parents wear reading glasses, no glaucoma, cataracts or macular degeneration in the family"
General Health	"I'm fit and well, with no health complaints, no diabetes or blood pressure problems"
Medication	"I'm not taking anything"
Allergies	"I'm not allergic to anything"
Family General Health	"All seem well, no health complaints, no diabetes, no strokes, no cancer or anything like that"
Hobbies/Interests	"Hiking, fine dining and socialising with friends"
Driving Status	"I drive a car - I don't need glasses to do so either"
Smoke / Drink	"I don't smoke, but do have thee odd glass of wine when dining"
VDU Use	"My job is computer heavy - I must use it about 10 hours a day"
Contact Lenses	"Never worn any - I don't feel I need glasses, so have never considered them"

Reflections on Case #001

David's case sounds very much like a routine eye examination. He is responding to a recall letter, meaning he is likely only attending because he has been reminded that routine eye examinations are important to monitor visual and eye health.

He has no presenting concerns and no symptoms, so he is a perfect candidate to work through a standard eye care routine with, without any specific additional tests or investigations required to provide solutions to any problems he is having. Obviously, if routine examination reveals something during the check up, this would require further investigation; although it is less likely to appear given this particular case history.

There are several points of interest in the case history that can provide discussion points in your management, should no abnormalities be detected upon testing.

VDU Use

David's role as an IT consultant sees him using the computer for prolonged periods of time. Be sure to discuss regular screen breaks, remembering to blink and to remain hydrated throughout the day.

UV Protection

He also notes he has hiking as his main hobby. Consider discussing where he likes to hike and whether or not he uses sunglasses. If he spends prolonged periods of time outdoors, he is exposing his eyes to the ultraviolet light of the sun and as such increasing his risk factors for basal cell carcinomas around the eye, cataracts and macular degeneration.

Discussing sunglasses with him educate him further on the importance of UV protection, whilst opening up a potential dispensing opportunity should the eye test result in no optical prescription being required.

Recall

Should all the findings of the eye examination be normal, with no concerns on his eye health, you should advise him that you will recall him for his next eye examination in 2 years*. You can advise him that if he feels his vision changes before then, he can contact us for advice sooner.

*Please note: recalls depend on numerous factors and this is a suggestion based on recommended recall dates and the patient having no findings or risk factors that warrant a shorter recall. Practitioner discretion is advised.

Case #002: Charlotte

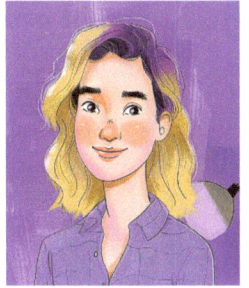

Composition – For the person acting as this patient:

Charlotte is a 27-year-old **student nurse**. She is helpful, friendly, and pleased to be fitted in for an eye examination today, as she struggles to get time off between lectures and placements. Charlotte provides information easily and answers are generally free-flowing upon questioning.

The blue text provides an example of the type of response you should provide to this question

Reason for Visit	"I'm here because you sent me a letter to say I am due an eye examination"
Last Eye Examination	"2 years ago - here"
Subjective Visual Assessment	"I'm not noticing any problems, distance, near and intermediate vision is fine. I don't need any glasses to help me see"
Key Symptoms	"No symptoms for me!" (No to any red flag questions asked)
LOFTSEA	N/A (as no symptoms to investigate)
Ocular History	"None - I've never worn glasses, no injuries, no eye diseases, no hospital visits. No eye issues at all."
Family Ocular History	"I've no significant eye problems. My parents wear reading glasses, no glaucoma, cataracts or macular degeneration in the family"
General Health	"I'm healthy, no health complaints like diabetes or blood pressure problems, or anything like that. I'm also not pregnant or breast feeding"
Medication	"I'm on the contraceptive pill and carry an epipen"
Allergies	"I'm VERY allergic to peanuts"
Family General Health	"All seem well, no health complaints, no diabetes, no strokes, no cancer or anything like that"
Hobbies/Interests	"Writing blogs, enjoys watching reality TV, plays on the university netball team"
Driving Status	"I drive a car to my lectures, that's about it"
Smoke / Drink	"I don't smoke but enjoy a drink at my netball socials!"
VDU Use	"It can vary. Most days 4 hours a day for university work, some days without as on placements"
Contact Lenses	"Never worn any - I don't need glasses, so I've never considered them"

Reflections on Case #002

Charlotte's case sounds very much like a routine eye examination. She is responding to a recall letter, meaning she is likely only attending because she has been reminded that routine eye examinations are important to monitor visual and eye health.

She has no presenting concerns and no symptoms, so she is a perfect candidate to work through a standard eye care routine with, without any specific additional tests or investigations required to provide solutions to any problems he is having. Obviously, if routine examination reveals something during the check up, this would require further investigation; although it is less likely to appear given this particular case history.

There are several points of interest in the case history that should be noted and understood. They may also contribute to Charlotte's management plan.

VDU Use
Charlotte's role as a student nurse sees her using the computer for prolonged periods of time on most days. Be sure to discuss regular screen breaks, remembering to blink and to remain hydrated throughout the day.

Allergies
Charlotte states that she is allergic to peanuts and carries an epipen. Whilst this may not fall into management advice, it is important to understand the extent of an allergy and record appropriately. I personally avoid any foods and fragrances that can trigger allergic responses in people and recommend avoiding peanuts (and other nut-based/nut-containing products) during breaks and lunch.

Contraceptive Pill
The contraceptive pill is often not disclosed during medication reviews. When wording your medication question, make reference to tablets/medicines or pills to prompt self-declaration, or you can ask directly (although this can be quite awkward). The contraceptive pill can cause symptoms of dry eye, blurring and epiphora (watering), so it is a useful medication to know a patient is taking when investigating these symptoms.

Recall
Should all the findings of the eye examination be normal, with no concerns on her eye health, you should advise her that you will recall her for her next eye examination in 2 years*. You can advise her that if she feels her vision changes before then, she can contact us for advice sooner.

*Please note: recalls depend on numerous factors and this is a suggestion based on recommended recall dates and the patient having no findings or risk factors that warrant a shorter recall. Practitioner discretion is advised.

Case #003: Eshika

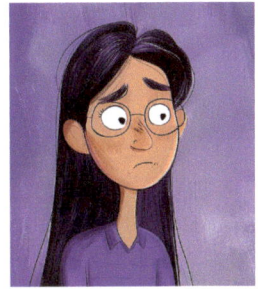

Composition – For the person acting as this patient:

Eshika is a 22-year-old trainee barista. She is anxious. She doesn't enjoy medical appointments, nor being asked questions. She gives minimal information away unless asked for it specifically and doesn't elaborate or divulge further information unless probed further.

Reveal only bold & purple text when asked but when probed further, add detail from non-bold text

Reason for Visit	"I need new glasses" (Current ones scratched and scratches obstruct vision)
Last Eye Examination	"Not too sure" (If pressed, say about 2 years ago)
Subjective Visual Assessment	"Scratch in my lens makes it hard to see at all distances" (If the scratch wasn't there, distance and near all clear)
Key Symptoms	"I'm not having any symptoms" (No to any red flag questions asked)
LOFTSEA	N/A (as no symptoms to investigate)
Ocular History	"I have stigmatisms" (Clarify it's astigmatism, also short sighted and worn glasses since age of 13. No hospital visits or other significant history)
Family Ocular History	"Mum and dad wear glasses" (Both are short-sighted, no eye diseases known)
General Health	"I am ok" (Being treated for anxiety. No other health issues, not pregnant)
Medication	"Sertraline"
Allergies	"Just hayfever"
Family General Health	"Mum has diabetes. Dad had a heart attack, and grandfather had a stroke"
Hobbies/Interests	"Going to the cinema, knitting club"
Driving Status	"I'm learning to drive" (Wears glasses during driving lessons)
Smoke / Drink	"I don't drink or smoke"
VDU Use	"I use it for Instagram and TikTok. Just on my phone"
Contact Lenses	"I'm scared to try them in case they get stuck around the back of my eye. It'd be nice not to wear glasses though…"

Reflections on Case #003

Eshika's case sounds very much like a routine eye examination and she is mainly attending as she has scratched glasses and is due an eye examination to re-authorise an optical prescription to buy them.

She has no significant presenting concerns and her vision seems stable, albeit from the scratched lens that will need replacing. Her age and history suggest minimal abnormalities will be found and a standard eye examination should be conducted to rule out any underlying issues.

There are several points of interest in the case history that should be noted and understood. They may also contribute to Eshika's management plan.

Anxiety

Eshika presents with an anxious demeanour and also states in her case history that she suffers from symptoms of anxiety. Her medication, sertraline, also shows that she is being treated for it. Approach the appointment in a gentle manner and reassure her frequently as you progress. You may need to limit your questions to seek the most essential information and respect her comfort level on what she is willing to divulge.

Scratched Lenses

Eshika's main reason for visit was the scratched lens on her glasses. Further prompting during the case history revealed potential lack of care of glasses. A gentle reassurance of keeping lenses away from surfaces, keeping the glasses in their case when not used and general lens care will help prevent this in the future. Additionally, she is likely to require a dispense, so be sure to advise on lens options before handing over to the dispensing team.

Contact Lenses

Eshika is open to the idea of contact lenses and, if asked, would have expressed an interest in them. She does have concerns they'd get stuck behind her eye, which as you know, is not a possibility - so gentle discussion and reassurance could open up the potential of a contact lens fit. These discussions help the patient, but also demonstrate you are commercially aware to practice owners and managers.

Recall

Should all the findings of the eye examination be normal, with no concerns on her eye health (or significant changes in her optical prescription), you should advise her that you will recall her for her next eye examination in 2 years. You can advise her that if she feels her vision changes before then, she can contact us for advice sooner.

Case #004: Desmond

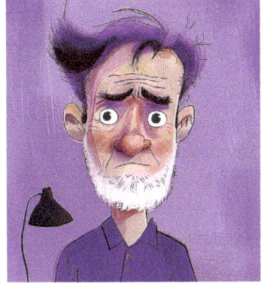

Composition – For the person acting as this patient:

Desmond is a 63-year-old **warehouse operative**, who is grumpy and combatant. He is difficult to obtain information from and requires careful wording of questions as to not anger him. He will often reply that he is in a rush, feels like being at the appointment is a waste of time and that answers to all questions "should be written down already". If calmed and reasoned with, he does calm and provide answers in a more relaxed matter.

The red text provides an example of the type of response you should provide to this question
(Smaller text in parenthesis to be used if probed appropriately and/or has managed to build rapport with Desmond)

Reason for Visit	"You tell me, you sent for me" (when asked to elaborate, say that a reminder came through the post)
Last Eye Examination	"You tell me" (2 years ago, here)
Subjective Visual Assessment	"I'm only here because you sent for me. I'd have told you if I had a problem, wouldn't I?"" (No problems, distance, intermediate and near vision fine)
Key Symptoms	"I've said my vision is fine!! Why so many darn questions?" (No red flag symptoms if asked)
LOFTSEA	N/A (as no symptoms to investigate)
Ocular History	"Just these plus two-hundreds from the pound store. You rip us off with those glasses out there!" (NV ok with +2.00 ready readers . No eye hospital visits, no eye diseases diagnosed)
Family Ocular History	"Me ma had glaucoma, but that should be written down already!" (Mother glaucoma -treatment and age of diagnosis unknown, no macular degeneration, no cataracts known)
General Health	"Why do you need to know about all that? It's rather personal, isn't it?" (Hypertension, high cholesterol, told at risk of stroke. No diabetes)
Medication	"Same as last time! It should be written down already!" (Simvastatin, Bendroflumethiazide, ramipril, atenolol)
Allergies	"Work" (Establish it was a joke - but no actual allergies)
Family General Health	"Same as last time! It should be written down already!" (No diabetes, grandfather had heart issues, sister has anaemia)
Hobbies/Interests	"Why do you need to know all this? What was the point of GDPR?" (Used to be a boxer, now coaches at local gym in spare time)
Driving Status	"Yeah, I drive. Doesn't everyone?"
Smoke / Drink	"What I do in my own time is my own business!" (Smokes 5 cigarettes a day maximum / a beer every evening)
VDU Use	"I don't deal with that rubbish" (No VDU use at all)
Contact Lenses	"What else are you trying to sell me?!" (Not interested)

Reflections on Case #004

Desmond's appointment, despite the confrontational nature of his history and symptoms, is another presentation of a routine eye examination, with special attention being needed to assess his eyes for the presence of glaucoma. Therefore at the end of the history, you should be considering a visual fields assessment, intraocular pressures measurement, full assessment of the optic nerve head and anterior chamber, with an OCT scan if available.

There were some areas of his history that would have made it difficult or uncomfortable to probe answers for, but would have been necessary to do so in order to best help him and his needs. If tackled appropriately, Desmond does provide the answers and his guard does drop. Ways that you can tackle patients like this can include:

 Remain calm: Whilst patients like this can make you feel threatened, remain calm and try not to panic.

 Explain: Take time to explain why you are asking these questions, showing empathy towards their reasons as to why the questions may feel invasive.

 Acknowledge their feelings: Many patients that present like this often have an underlying reason for it. They may be anxious, they may be concerned you will find something wrong or may have been wronged by a healthcare professional before. If safe to do so, seek to understand why they are being confrontational.

 Avoid confrontation: It can be difficult not to get defensive or tackle these encounters with higher energy than you are used to using. Maintain professionalism but also make it clear that mutual respect is needed in these situations

 Safety: In this case, Desmond was not going to be more than grumpy, obtuse or defensive, but if you ever feel that a situation is getting heated, do not be afraid to call for a colleague or exit the room for safety.

I know that I have said this in the bullet point directly above but:

If you ever feel unsafe, don't hesitate to step out and/or call for help!

I would also like to use this moment to point out that as optometrists, we are often in a position of lone working (i.e. we are working alone in a room with a member of the public). It has been established that this has inherent risks and as such all professionals should work with their employer(s) to understand their lone-worker policies to ensure that you are kept safe should a patient become threatening.

If your clinic testing room has been fitted with a panic button - then learn where it is, when to use it and what the protocol is when the button has been pressed. I have worked in over 50 testing rooms and have only encountered a panic button a handful of times - but be reassured, despite being in practice for over a decade, I have never needed to use one!

Returning to Desmond's case history, here are several points of interest within it that should be noted and understood. They may also contribute to Desmond's management plan.

Ready Readers

Desmond is using "plus two hundreds" for reading. You may find that similar terms are used by patients in practice when using over the counter products, but it is advisable to measure the glasses anyway (and in the case of ready readers, it should be easy to hand-neutralise with trial lenses to confirm their powers).

Your refraction of Desmond's eyes should provide you adequate understanding of his refractive needs, but generally speaking ready readers are not appropriate for prolonged use. Discussion about optimal prescriptive eyewear for his needs should be discussed.

Risk Factors

Desmond has risk factors for glaucoma. His most significant risk factor for glaucoma is a family history (his mother), but he also has hypertension. His previous hobby of boxing is likely to mean he has sustained a few punches to the eye, of which may also contribute to his glaucomatous risk factors. When risk factors for conditions are revealed in the case history, make sure you plan to investigate the associated condition further within your assessment and document positive and negative results.

Smoking Status

Desmond is a smoker. Smoking has long been established as a major modifiable risk factor for numerous eye diseases such as macular degeneration, cataracts and dry eye. Use this encounter, where you have built sufficiently enough rapport with Desmond, to advise him of the dangers that smoking pose to his eyes.

General Health

Desmond is not in the best of health and has been advised that he is hypertensive and has high cholesterol, which his doctor has informed him has put him at high risk of having a stroke. This would warrant you to spend extra attention when assessing his blood vessels during fundoscopy as these conditions can cause tortuosity and emboli, affecting the health of the retina.

Rip Off!

Desmond also states that glasses are a rip off and accuses us of trying to constantly sell him things when we mention contact lenses. There is a common misconception that optometrists and opticians are just salespeople (unfortunately the media and the public underfunding for eye services do not help with this). When patients challenge the sales side of the role, do not become defensive, explain the benefits of what you are selling and discuss alternative options.

With this book being written during a cost-of-living crisis, you will find many patients are avoiding unnecessary spending. Therefore, Desmond's attitude could be related to this. Be assertive with what costs are necessary and **NEVER** pressure a patient into an unnecessary sale.

Recall*

From the case history, it is hard to determine when you would expect to see him again as this will be highly dependent on the health of his eyes, in respect to his risk factors.

The minimum recall date for a patient with a family history of glaucoma, according the NHS eligibility, would be 12 months*, but the NHS advise against blanket minimum recall periods on each group, especially if there are no additional reasons to recall sooner than two years*.

Whilst it isn't possible to determine when you would need to see Desmond again from this history and symptoms, the internal monologuing about when you need to see him next should start when you are taking his history.

*Please note: recalls depend on numerous factors and this suggestion is based on recommended recall dates and the patient having no findings or risk factors that warrant a shorter recall. Practitioner discretion is advised.

Case #005: Annie

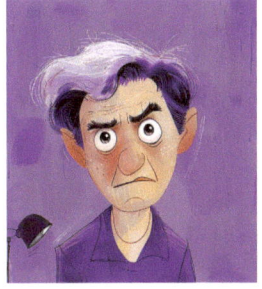

Composition – For the person acting as this patient:

Annie is a 72-year-old **retired nurse**, who is grumpy and combatant. She is difficult to obtain information from and requires careful wording of questions as to not anger her. She will often reply that she is in a rush, feel like being at the appointment is a waste of time and that answers to all questions "should be written down already". If calmed and reasoned with, she does calm and provide answers in a more relaxed matter.

The red text provides an example of the type of response you should provide to this question
(Smaller text in parenthesis to be used if probed appropriately and/or has managed to build rapport with Annie)

Reason for Visit	"Here because you called me to book in" (when asked to elaborate, say that a reminder came through the post)
Last Eye Examination	"Shouldn't be written down?" (2 years ago, here)
Subjective Visual Assessment	"Everything is fine. I can see stuff far away, also ok reading in my reading glasses" (No problems, distance, intermediate and near vision fine - with NV glasses)
Key Symptoms	"I've said my vision is fine! Are you not listening to me?" (No red flag questions upon questioning)
LOFTSEA	N/A (as no symptoms to investigate)
Ocular History	"I just wear the over the counter glasses - +2.75 I think. Surely the rest you should know, I've been coming here for decades!!" (NV ok with +2.75 ready readers. No eye hospital visits, no eye diseases)
Family Ocular History	"I was adopted, so I don't know anything about my family history"
General Health	"Dodgy heart, had a heart attack last year. I have atrial fibrillation and was told last week I was borderline diabetic. The joys of aging!"
Medication	"Too many to tell you, surely you should have a list!?" (press - bisoprolol, bendroflumethiazide, simvastatin, candesartan)
Allergies	"Cat hair"
Family General Health	"I mean you are clearly not listening to me. I've told you I am adopted!"
Hobbies/Interests	"Crochet, knitting, playing games on a tablet"
Driving Status	"Of course I drive a car. How else would I have gotten here?"
Smoke / Drink	"I don't smoke, but do drink red wine every Wednesday as a treat"
VDU Use	"Haven't got time for that!" (Uses phone to check emails and Facebook)
Contact Lenses	"Why on earth would I want them?" (Not interested)

Reflections on Case #005

Annie's case history is another routine presentation, again, with a quite fierce undertone. She presents for a routine eye examination and, with little family history and lack of symptoms, there may be little to suggest that further investigation is required, unless something reveals itself as an incidental finding during her examination.

There are several points of interest in the case history that should be noted and understood. They may also contribute to Annie's management plan. Some areas of interest may be duplicate of previous cases. As such, from here, I will highlight case-specific observations that may not have been covered on previous cases.

Adopted

Annie informs us that she is adopted. In many cases of adoption, there is little information on family history and as such prevents us with a stumbling block when addressing inherited risk factors.

It is to be noted that there are two parts of the case history that require asking about family health, so do keep in mind what a patient has already revealed. A person who says they never knew their parents due to adoption and don't know if they had any eye diseases are not going to be "un-adopted" by the time you come around to asking about family health issues. Use common sense and be sensitive around this issue - else you may encounter comments very similar to Annie's if you did ask about family history twice!

"See Previous"

Annie is quite abrupt when we ask her about her medications and tells us that it should already be noted down. However, her general health has changed dramatically since the time you saw her 2 years ago; having had the heart attack last year and is now considered to be pre-diabetic.

The medication she does reveal to be taking look geared towards her heart. These medications are likely to have been adjusted since you saw her last, with new ones added. So even if you do get the "it should be written down" line from a patient, don't be tempted to write "see previous" or copy and paste the last entry without checking - as you may very well record it incorrectly!

Case #006: Adnan

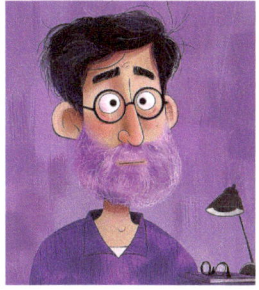

Composition – For the person acting as this patient:

Adnan is a 60-year-old translator and does not reveal information easily. He only answers directly to what is being asked and offers no more information. If you are asked a question, do answer honestly but don't give more information than what is being asked, nor provide any additional context.

Reveal only bold & purple text when asked **but when probed further, add detail from non-bold text**

Reason for Visit	"Overdue an eye examination"
Last Eye Examination	"4 years ago" (Did have many reminders over last few months)
Subjective Visual Assessment	"It's ok" (Needs varifocals for all distances now, but vision fine with them)
Key Symptoms	"None" (No red flag symptoms on questioning)
LOFTSEA	N/A (as no symptoms to investigate)
Ocular History	"Yeah, it's fine" (Wears varifocals, had a retinal detachment about 6 years ago, think was the left eye. Aware has a cataract forming in the left eye)
Family Ocular History	"Dad has glaucoma" (Father has glaucoma, uses drops. Aged 70 at time of diagnosis. No other family history of eye diseases)
General Health	"It's ok" (No diabetes, no blood pressure issues. Possibly a bit overweight)
Medication	"Yeah I do" (Need to press - omeprazole as occasionally gets acid reflux)
Allergies	"Some antibiotics" (Amoxicillin and other penicillin-based ones)
Family General Health	"Don't know, parents are dead now" (Father died of a stroke. Mother died of heart attack)
Hobbies/Interests	"Travelling. Writing a travel blog"
Driving Status	"Yeah, I drive" (Car. Also has HGV license. Wears glasses to drive)
Smoke / Drink	"No, I don't smoke or drink"
VDU Use	"Yeah I use a computer" (High usage – 6 hours a day. Mainly for work but occasionally for writing a blog. Work use is a desktop and writes blog on a laptop)
Contact Lenses	"No thanks" (Not interested - has a phobia about things going near eyes)

Reflections on Case #006

Adnan is a very reserved character and doesn't offer much in response to our questions. There may be many reasons behind this, ranging from being shy or anxious to not being interested in being at the appointment and having his mind elsewhere. It is not for us to pry into this, but efforts must be taken to probe for further information to ensure the case history is as complete as it needs to be in order to conduct his eye examination.

There are several points of interest in the case history that should be noted and understood. They may also contribute to Adnan's management plan. Some areas of interest may be duplicate of previous cases. As such, from here, I will highlight case-specific observations that may not have been covered on previous cases.

Short Responses

Adnan is quick to say everything is fine and ok and, in many parts of the history, this is correct and to the point. However, there are areas where these short answers aren't wholly correct.

Upon probing his ocular history, it is revealed that he has had a retinal detachment in the past. This may explain the presence of scarring in the eye when you examine him; else it would be something of a mystery upon discovering it.

Just taking these short answer responses may seem good and allow you to fly through the history and symptoms quickly, but care must be taken to ensure you have as much relevant information as you need to be safe and to advise appropriately.

Areas of potential missed information in this case include: ocular health, general health, medications, allergies, family general health. VDU usage and the types of vehicle he drives.

"They're All Dead"

Despite the dramatic subheading here, I have found that a lot of patients reply with words along these lines when asking about family histories. When probing, you find out that they all died of heart failure, or strokes, or other significant health conditions.

Don't take "they are all dead now" as an answer to family health without probing. Just because the relative has died, doesn't remove that risk factor you are looking for.

That said, be empathetic and sensitive around this subject as grief can manifest in many different ways and asking around this topic can upset your patient.

Case #007: Jonathan

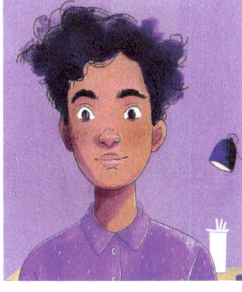

Composition – For the person acting as this patient:

Jonathan is a very chatty, 33-year old **data administrator**. Talk excessively when answering the questions and feel free to ad-lib if you want to go away from the suggested text in green. If the practitioner tries to bring you back on track, do follow their guidance and give the answer in black, but as soon as they allow you free-roam to answer, take the opportunity to excessively talk. Please note this script covers several pages.

The green text provides an example of the type of response you should provide to this question
(Smaller text in parenthesis to be used if the practitioner brings Jonathan and his excessive talking under control)

Reason for Visit	"Well, see I set up my Alexa to remind me that I need to have an eye examination every 2 years at the last appointment I had. You know, Alexa?? Really useful they are. Anyway, it reminded me on Tuesday last week that I was due for my 2-year eye examination and that is why I booked one." (due check up)
Last Eye Examination	"Oh it was at the time that you had that lovely gentleman Alex on the front desk. He sorted out my sunglasses lovely last time. I was sad as he said he was leaving that day to go and study that eye thing, um, yes, optometrically or opticianry, yes. How is he? Are you going to offer him a job at the end of his studies?" (2 years ago, here)
Subjective Visual Assessment	"I am so glad you asked, I was watching the television the other day and wondered what was going on. I usually have the subtitles on but silly me, realised that I didn't have them on, so wasn't able to read them! I'd struggle if they let me loose out in the real world, I really would. I mean when I found the button to turn them on, I was fine but phew, I was worried for a bit there. I also couldn't read my phone the other day but think that was because I had the brightness set to a minimum…" (No problems, distance, intermediate and near all fine)
Key Symptoms	Say "No" to every question but follow with "What is that?" (No red flag symptoms on questioning)
LOFTSEA	N/A (as no symptoms to investigate)
Ocular History	"I love this question as it reminds me of that time I bought a pair of glasses at the pound store. I put them on but couldn't see very far away so figured they made the glasses wrong. Oh and then I had that trip to the local eye hospital place for retinal surgery. Wait, that wasn't me, that was for my neighbour." (No glasses, no ocular history, no trips to the eye hospital)
Family Ocular History	"Everyone in my family wears glasses. I don't know what for but they always have done. I particularly like my uncle's glasses. Oh, you mean eye diseases? Well, my wife recently got diagnosed with high pressure in her eyes." (No significant family ocular history, no glaucoma)

General Health	"I'm a little overweight. I had a cold a few weeks ago and COVID-19 back in 2020. That was rough. I was unwell for weeks and could barely move. Anyway, glad that is over with now. I thankfully haven't seen the doctor for years. He isn't keen on seeing me for some reason." (No significant general health issues, no diabetes, no hypertension)
Medication	"What do you mean by medication? I take a vitamin pill every morning and then the occasional paracetamol if I get a headache ot hurt my back. I don't think I take anything from the doctor, that said, he really doesn't like seeing me so I guess I might need medication. Do you think I might need medication then?" (No medication)
Allergies	"I don't particularly like salad dressing, it really doesn't agree with my stomach. I don't think it is allergies per se, but I think the taste is awful and really I don't like the texture. Oh – you mean like stuff that triggers me to have an actual allergy? None at all. Thankfully!" (No allergies)
Family General Health	"Well mum is currently off work with a cold. She had a fall a few years back too. They say she has diabetes too. Bless her. My dad is being treated for prostate cancer but I am unsure what that has to do with me. Will I have these conditions too? Is that why you are asking about them?" (Mother has diabetes, Father has prostate cancer)
Hobbies/Interests	"I'd be lost without my game consoles. Love them. I had the very first Pokemon game and never looked back. Did you know In the beta version of Pokemon Red & Blue, Koffing and Weezing were originally named Ny and La respectively. These names were references to New York City and Los Angeles, two large cities that are associated with heavy pollution. Cool, isn't it?" (Videogames, internet chat forums, politics)
Driving Status	"Me? Behind the wheel of a car? No thank you. Never have driven and never will. Far too much pollution for my liking. I mean, the bike is good enough for me. I get everywhere by bike you know. See that green one over the road attached to the railings? That one is mine. It set me back a pretty penny mind you!" (Non-driver)
Smoke / Drink	"Both are not habits I wish to engage in. Lost a friend of mine to smoking. Terrible shame. He smoked 40 a day and he ended getting some form of cancer. I'm also not the biggest fan of drinking. I had way to much Southern Comfort on my 19th birthday and that's put me off the stuff for life!" (No / No)
VDU Use	"I don't think there is a time that I am not on the computer. I am always using a screen. Or do you just mean like a desktop. Or laptop? Or do you mean VDU screens of any type? I am constantly looking at a screen though. Perhaps not now but I see your sight chart is on a screen so I guess I am using one now…" (High usage: 8+ hours a day)
Contact Lenses	"Why would I ever want to stick plastic in my eye? No thanks!" (Not interested)

Reflections on Case #007

Jonathan is very pleasant, albeit chatty patient that has the need to chat to you as a practitioner. Whilst this level of chattiness is extreme, it does demonstrate that patients can gain control over a conversation if you don't set the pace and the tone. Patients such as Jonathan do exist and as such you will need to find ways to keep that control.

There are several points of interest in the case history that should be noted and understood. They may also contribute to Jonathan's management plan. Some areas of interest may be duplicate of previous cases. As such, from here, I will highlight case-specific observations that may not have been covered on previous cases.

Engagement

Jonathan will need to be engaged throughout the appointment and will require many gentle nudges to stay on track. His need to communicate will need to be considered when examining him and as such you will need to be aware of ways that talking will impede the flow of your routine.

Very Little From a Lot of Talking

You will have noticed that Jonathan says very little of clinical value compared to the number of words he uses. You will need to make a conscious effort to pick the information that is relevant from the discussion and then hone in with closed questions to clarify key points. You may also opt to ask fewer open questions in this case, as this could mean further opportunities for Jonathan to control the conversation.

Time Management

Some patients that are similar to Jonathan are fascinating to talk to. They may discuss their interesting hobbies, the amazing feats that they have accomplished or just have lived a wholesome life with lots of stories. Whilst it is good to use this as a chance to build rapport, you need to remember that you are there to perform an eye examination and that you have an appointment diary to keep to.

Ways to still have these meaningful conversations without overrunning often include continuing with the eye examination and letting them talk during moments that you are recording data or setting up equipment. This works well as it assists with the patient's need to communicate, avoids the awkward silences as you complete your records and still shows that you are interested in them as a person.

Gentle Interruptions

There may be times where you do need to gain control of the appointment again and there is nothing wrong in providing a gentle interruption and guiding the talk back to the eye examination.

An example of what I have used is:

> *"...and that's really interesting! But if we could get back to the eye examination right now and we can continue in just a moment."*

This polite, but direct, interruption can help steer the conversation back to the reason they are here, but also make them feel that you are still interested, often with the expectation they will be allowed to continue shortly. These statements are particularly impactful if you are about to change topic.

Keeping it in the Family

You may have caught Jonathan mentioning his wife in the section about family ocular health. Patients mentioning significant others and family members by marriage (e.g. brother-in-law or sister-in-law) having ocular or general health problems in response to this question happens regularly.

Be mindful that this is not relevant information to the appointment, but do display empathy at the news. Don't challenge or tell the patient it isn't relevant as this could be perceived as rude, uncaring or standoffish, but you can move the conversation on towards more relevant, blood-relatives.

Clarify and Consolidate

Clarify points that you are uncertain of. Patients that talk excessively can be overwhelming as they can provide many points you need to investigate in a short space of time. Try to consolidate what they have said, clarify any points you are uncertain of and make sure you address their key concerns.

VDU Use

Jonathan has stated he uses a screen excessively. Use this as a discussion point in the management to encourage him to blink regularly, take regular breaks from the screens and to stay hydrated.

You may wish to examine his eyes for signs of dry eye or investigate his accommodation - especially if he has mentioned symptoms of eyestrain.

Closing Notes on Case Study Selection 1

This case study selection focused on patients that have attended for a routine eye examination with minimal symptoms or concerns. These patients will make up the majority of your patients in clinic, should you choose to work in a high-street opticians utilising a standard primary care optometry model.

Whilst it may seem that there is little to be concerned about on their initial presentations, there can be real benefit from taking the time to conduct a thorough case-history. Let us explore them below.

Reason for Visit	By understanding their reason for visit, you can identify what type of eye examination you will conduct. As you have seen from case studies 001 - 007, they have all attended and stated they are generally happy with their vision and have no concerns, so a straightforward routine test can be planned for.
Family Clues	Finding out about the patient's family history may highlight areas where you need to deviate from the standard assessment and perform additional tests. An example of this are the cases where there is a family history of glaucoma, where you'll need to adapt your routine to include further investigations into assessing their risk of developing glaucoma.
Glasses Talk	Some patients don't require glasses, but keen discussion around additional eyewear needs (such as sunglasses or safety glasses) will help educate the patient on eye care and potentially open up an avenue for a dispense. Furthermore, those that use "off-the-peg" ready-readers would benefit the discussion on how they are a "one-size-fits-all" and doesn't account for key individual factors such as astigmatism correction, anisometropia or pupillary distances - which can subsequently lead to symptoms of eyestrain and blurring.
Contact Lenses	All of the patients in this first selection of case histories did not wear contact lenses. It is always wise to ask about them as some may be suitable candidates to fit - both offering your patient an additional way to correct their optical prescription and the practice to source another stream of income. Those patients that do not have a prescription are also worth mentioning contact lenses to - not to prescribe them per se, but to see if they are using unlicensed cosmetic lenses and to discuss the risks of using them.

Personalities	This selection of case histories demonstrated a handful of the types of patients that you will see in your clinics. Some will be easy to get along with and comply with questioning and procedures with minimal issue. Some will be anxious, shy or combatant and as such you will need to be able to adapt to their way of being assessed (within reason!) to best obtain the most relevant information from them.
Information Expectations	Some patients might think all eye practices and health clinics have all of their information. They may believe the previous eye professional they saw had perfectly recorded all of the information they provided (from experience, this is sadly not the case!) If you don't have some details, ask them. Explain why it's important. If they think you should already know, gently ask why they think that – sometimes, there's confusion or misinformation over their expectation. Being open and honest with them can often de-escalate an issue before it becomes one!
Emotions	Patients can sometimes be upset or angry. Take a moment to figure out why. It's likely not your fault (unless you did kept them waiting too long or addressed them by the wrong name!). Their emotions may have basis in anxiety, fear, or frustration. Understanding where their feelings come from helps you address things carefully and build their trust.

That said, keep in mind a message I have pressed earlier in this chapter:

If you ever feel unsafe, don't hesitate to remove yourself from the situation and/or call for help!

In a nutshell, these routine eye examinations are more than just a check-up. They're opportunities to connect with patients, even if they don't have many concerns upfront. A good chat about their history can uncover important info and set the stage for providing them the best eye care.

Case Study Selection 2

Visual Concerns

This chapter provides examples of patients presenting with visual difficulties – from the gradual difficulties with reading associated to presbyopia to the sudden loss of vision in an eye.

You may encounter these scenarios regularly in extended/enhanced services such as **MECS** (Minor Eye Care Scheme) or **CUES** (Coronavirus Urgent Eye Service) style appointments, but they do crop up in routine clinics. Therefore, it is essential that you know how to thoroughly investigate the potential causes and by taking a thorough case history, you will be able to efficiently identify the relevant tests to perform to get to a tentative diagnosis promptly.

As you progress through these case histories, you will develop your way of navigating visual difficulties and concerns, prompting you to identify the likely causes of vision loss early on and, as such, allow you to select the most appropriate tests to make efficient use of your appointment time. The cases are also written to include several risk factors for pathology, so being able to identify the risk factors among the presenting symptoms will further your knowledge and understanding.

Please remember that all of the following cases are fictional patients, but representing real-world presentations. Any similarities to people, real or fictional, is purely co-incidental.

Case #008: Shelly

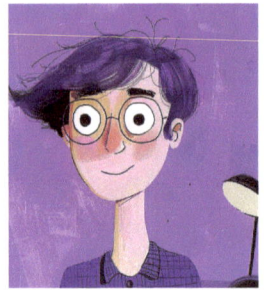

Composition – For the person acting as this patient:

Shelly is a very anxious 45-year-old **magazine editor**. She is relieved to be fitted into your diary, but has been waiting for an appointment for over a month and is very concerned that her symptoms are serious. She is not quick to give answers to questions and you may need to build rapport with the practitioner to open up.

Reveal only bold & purple text when asked but when probed further, add detail from non-bold text

Please note that this script spans two pages due to the introduction of the "LOFTSEA" section.

Reason for Visit	"Can't see up close very well. Needed an urgent appointment to see if anything serious"
Last Eye Examination	"4 years ago" (at "Eyeglass and Lens" Opticians)
Subjective Visual Assessment	"Near vision is terrible" Distance is ok, intermediate vision is ok-ish but harder to keep focus
Key Symptoms	"Near vision is terrible" (poor near vision but no flashes, no floaters, no pain, no redness, no light sensitivity, no diplopia and no headaches)
LOFTSEA	
Location	"Both eyes"
Onset	"About a month - booked to see you ASAP but this was the first appointment that you had!" (gradual decrease in near vision, has been having diffiuculties adjusting to different distances for about 6 months
Frequency	"Any time I look at something close"
Type	"Blurring of vision at near"
Self Treatment	"Holding things further away helps" (finding arms are not long enough!)
Effect on Life	"Significant. I can't see to work properly!" (worried about meeting deadlines and worried about losing job if can't see. Additionally worried going blind)
Associated	"Eyes feel really tired after a long day"

Ocular History	**"I wear glasses and have done since I was 12"** (Wears single vision distance glasses, was told was long-sighted. No trips eye hospital visits. Had a case of bacterial conjunctivitis 6 years ago - all resolved. No eye diseases)
Family Ocular History	**"My grandmother had cataracts in her eyes"** (No other family ocular history, no known glaucoma or macular disease)
General Health	**"I'm ok"** (Anxiety. No diabetes, no hypertension/other health issues. Not pregnant/breastfeeding)
Medication	**"Yeah, one for my anxiety"** (Need to ask specifically which one: citalopram)
Allergies	**"Latex and sticking plasters"**
Family General Health	**"My grandad died of oesophageal cancer"** (Mother has diabetes, sister recent hip operation)
Hobbies/Interests	**"Reading"** (If made to feel comfortable: has won local pub quiz the most times)
Driving Status	**"I drive"** (Car. Wears glasses. Has no problems with vision when driving but noticing the dashboard is a little more difficult of late)
Smoke / Drink	**"I don't smoke. I occasionally have a glass of gin at a special event"**
VDU Use	**"You'd have thought that being an editor, I'd be a computer user!"** (High usage – approximately 8 hours a day. Work use only - desktop)
Contact Lenses	**"Never really considered them as nobody has ever suggested them to me"** (Could be interested if would solve the issue of changing from distance to near. Ask a few questions to the practitioner to see what they suggest)

Reflections on Case #008
Tentative Diagnosis: Presbyopia

Shelly has presented with concerns of reduced near vision, which is typical of a patient presenting with reduced near vision at this age. She is clearly anxious and there is a potential for her to be aggravated due to the delay in seeing her. This may be compounded by the role she has as a magazine editor, of which I have heard from several patients is a very stressful role.

There are several points of interest in the case history that should be noted and understood. They may also contribute to Shelly's management plan. Some areas of interest may be duplicate of previous cases. As such, I will highlight case-specific observations that may not have been covered on previous cases.

Empathy

Shelly is anxious about her reduced vision and the concerns it has on her ability to work to the strict deadlines of her job. For optometrists seeing patients with presbyopia, we know that this is a normal change associated with age and can be easily rectified by introducing a near prescription. For our patients, they are not likely to encounter these symptoms or know what they are caused by until they become presbyopic and as such can be a very worrying time for them - especially if they have never experienced problems with their eyes before or have never worn glasses. Whilst it may be a common and simple optometric problem for us - it will likely be a big deal for your patient - so be empathetic!

I often talk to my patients on the verge of becoming presbyopia around the time of their next eye examination and advise them of the likelihood that their near vision will deteriorate within the next 2-5 years and reassure them that it is a normal change, but to have it looked into should it start to affect their day to day life.

LOFTSEA

Shelly's presentation introduces us to the first patient with symptoms and as such, the symptoms should be investigated with the LOFTSEA questions. With these questions, you can see how much more information you can learn from the patient's symptoms and identify how significant they are.

It's important to recognise that the depth of questioning shouldn't be limited to the main LOFTSEA questions. A deeper exploration within these areas can reveal additional insights into the onset of the patient's symptoms and their broader impact on daily life. However, it's crucial to remember that a patient who has been reserved in their responses is likely to remain so, even when asked about the specifics of LOFTSEA.

Visual Correction

Whilst this case demonstrates just the case history, the presentation and the answers to the questions, especially those from LOFTSEA, would provide a tentative diagnosis of presbyopia. You would need to run the full routine to assess her visual status and refractive requirements, but you would also use this time to think about discussions around likely optical correction.

In this case, presbyopia was the diagnosis and as such a reading prescription was issued, alongside her distance prescription. You would need to factor in time within the management to discuss ways to dispense the prescription (including the pros and cons of each). This could include:

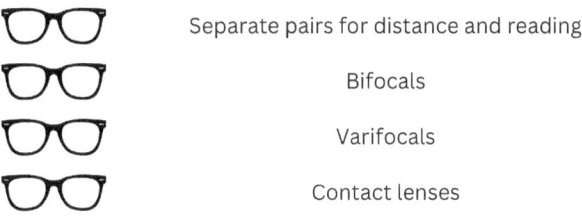

Separate pairs for distance and reading

Bifocals

Varifocals

Contact lenses

Contact Lenses

Shelly states that she has never been talked to regarding contact lenses. It may be that the previous practitioner did not feel that she was a good candidate for them, so never discussed them, or she may have forgotten that she has been asked. Additionally, she may think that it won't be suitable for her as she needs two corrections (one for distance and one for near) and as such may not have considered them going forward, unless you would have asked.

If a patient expresses interest, be sure to investigate further their needs and wants - remember, contact lens technology is progressing at a rapid pace and there is now a lens available for most patients. Multifocals, monovision or correction for distance with the option of reading glasses over the top - there are modes of correcting visual prescriptions that also will suit most people. Make sure you ask and make sure you find out more!

"One for my…"

Shelly is taking medication but has said it is "one for my". Patients may not instantly say what medication they are taking or expect you to know the medication is based on the condition. Whilst you will identify many conditions based on the medication they are taking, be sure to press and clarify so you can record appropriately. Shelly does reveal she is taking citalopram upon asking.

Some may have things written down or even bring in a copy of their latest prescription receipt. To aid time, you could also ask your reception team to request patients bring copies or lists of their medications at time of booking.

Case #009: Royston

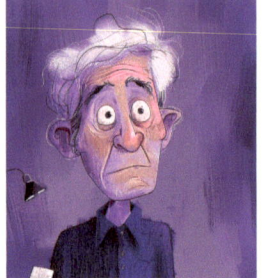

Composition – For the person acting as this patient:

Royston is an 85-year-old retired male. He is very concerned about his symptoms and will constantly ask if he is going blind throughout the appointment. Try and push for an answer to this question, but if the person taking the case history manages to explain that they will be unable to give you a clear answer until they have taken your history and investigated the symptoms, ease up on pushing for an answer.

Reveal only bold & purple text when asked **but when probed further, add detail from non-bold text**
Please note that this script spans two pages due to the "LOFTSEA" section.

Reason for Visit	"I woke up this morning with a blob in the centre of my vision of my left eye. It's all wavy around it and I can't see well out of the eye at all. Have I gone blind?"
Last Eye Examination	"6 months ago - I think the lady at the front said I'm too early to be seen and have to pay for today. Is that right?"
Subjective Visual Assessment	"Terrible, I'm afraid. Left eye can't see well at all. My right eye seems ok though. Does this mean my left eye has gone blind? Will my right eye go blind too?"
Key Symptoms	"This new floaty blob in the left eye and waviness" (No other red flag symptoms on questioning)
LOFTSEA	
Location	"Left eye. I've said the left eye is the one causing the issue. right in the middle"
Onset	"This morning" (whilst sudden change today, the vision in the left eye has been deteriorating over a few years)
Frequency	"It's there all the time since it happened. I'm blind, aren't I?"
Type	"It's really bad in my left eye - can you tell me when it'll go?"
Self Treatment	"Nothing has helped so far" (if pressed, finds things easier to read if closes left eye and only uses the right eye)
Effect on Life	"I'm scared I'll never see well again! I'm going to have to give up my car! I love driving and my independence!"
Associated	"Seems like straight lines are wavy. It's that or I need a new doorframe at home!"

Ocular History	"I wear reading glasses, not that I can use them very well now I've just lost my sight in my left eye. I thought having both cataracts removed 10 years ago would mean I wouldn't have more eye problems again. Apparently I had dry eyes last time I was here? They never feel dry - I'm not sure I understood what the last person meant" (No glaucoma, no other eye issues)
Family Ocular History	"My mother had a macular - or something along those lines. I never really knew what it was" (No other family ocular history, no known glaucoma)
General Health	"They say I'm good for my age. Just got the blood pressure and my cholesterol is a little high. Is that why I am going blind?" (No diabetes, no other significant health issues)
Medication	"My wife would know. Can you ask her?" (see if practitioner prompts or helps identify a way to find out. If so: Atenolol, ramipril, simvastatin)
Allergies	"Nothing so far" (None)
Family General Health	"Me dad had a heart attack, and mum had the sugar" (Clarify that "had the sugar" means that she was diabetic)
Hobbies/Interests	"I like watching the football, used to go to watch but now only watch on the TV. Crosswords are ok - but I can't do that with my left eye being difficult!"
Driving Status	"My pride and joy is my Lotus Esprit, mainly drive for pleasure. I do have a little Hyundai that I drive to the shops. You're gonna tell me I can't do that now, aren't you? But I can see fine to drive!" (car driver - no distance glasses worn, drove to appointment today, despite vision issues.)
Smoke / Drink	"I quit last year. I was on 20 a day. For 65 years. I can't believe how much money I had wasted on that! Still have a couple of bitters at the social club each week though"
VDU Use	"Never touched one" (No use - has old non-smartphone for emergencies)
Contact Lenses	"Never needed distance glasses since my cataract ops - will they stop me going blind?" (Not really interested but if pushed, pursue action of how they would help with the vision in the left eye)

Reflections on Case #009

Tentative Diagnosis: Left Eye - Macular Disease - likely wet AMD

Royston has presented extremely worried that he has gone blind in his left eye, of which has caused him to push for an answer that you cannot yet provide him - has he gone blind in his left eye?

There are several points of interest in the case history that should be noted and understood. They may also contribute to Royston's management plan. Some areas of interest may be duplicate of previous cases. As such, I will highlight case-specific observations that may not have been covered on previous cases.

Sudden Vision Loss

A sudden loss of vision in one eye is something of an alarm bell to an optometrist seeing a patient. Often changes of a refractive nature are gradual and not-usually as drastic as causing significant vision loss. Whilst you should take every patient concern seriously, those presenting with significant symptoms warrant deeper questioning to tentatively diagnose, as so you can structure your investigations appropriately.

Demonstrate You Are Listening

As mentioned in an earlier chapter, you need to make sure that you are actively demonstrating that you are listening to your patient. Many practitioners fall into the trap of going through the motions of asking questions without taking note of what the patient is saying. This can be seen in this case study when we move on to the LOFTSEA questions.

Royston has stated several times that he is having problems in the LEFT eye and it is affecting the CENTRE of his vision. Therefore, you already have the answer to the "location" question of LOFTSEA and as such it does not need to be asked. That said, if you want to know more about the location (e.g is it at the top or bottom part of the vision), you can probe - but be sure to paraphrase what they have already said to make sure they know you are asking for more detail.

Has He Gone Blind?

A common question Royston is pushing is whether or not he has gone blind. You will often get these forward questions from patients and often the answer is not going to reveal itself until you have thoroughly investigated via taking their history and examining the patient. You need to let the patient know, empathetically, that you can't inform them appropriately until you have looked.

Be cautious that you do not appear to be dismissing their concerns, but also do not give false hope or confidence by saying "of course not" as your findings may indicate a diagnosis with a poor visual prognosis for the patient. Reassure them that you will do what you can to understand what is happening and that you will do your best to advise when you know more.

Previous History Helps

Royston states that he has been seen here before. This means you will have further information to help enlighten you of his ocular health on a record card. He commented that he had "dry eyes" last time and was confused by the diagnosis as he never had symptoms. He even admits that he didn't really understand what his last optometrist told him.

Given the symptoms present today and the mention of "dry" - would have me think of dry macular degeneration that has converted to wet macular degeneration and as such, plan my assessment to rule out this as the cause. His previous records (and photographs) indicated that he had significant drusen and dry macular degeneration last time, giving strength to our tentative diagnosis of wet AMD.

Risk Factors

Remember the reasons behind why you ask certain questions on the case history. It shouldn't be a case of going through the motions for an extra mark in an examination or asking because "that's what we do when we take history and symptoms".

Royston has significant risk factors for wet AMD.

- History of dry AMD
- Increased age
- Family history of AMD (likely mother had AMD from history)
- Hypertension
- High cholesterol
- History of being a heavy smoker

Whilst this is not an exhaustive list of AMD risk factors, Royston does have a large number of risk factors for the disease. This further adds strength to our tentative diagnosis.

Colloquialisms

Royston uses a few colloquialisms (a word or phrase that is not formal or literary and is used in ordinary or familiar conversation). His mother "had a macular" and "had the sugar".

Some are easy to understand (we all have maculas, but frequently seen people use the term "has the macular" to mean AMD) with others a little trickier ("has the sugar" has been known to be used to inappropriately refer to someone with type 2 diabetes) and as such you may need to ask further questions to clarify what they mean, or use them as educational moments for correct terminology.

"My Wife Would Know"

Often patients will not know what medication they are taking (as discussed in previous cases). Whilst some will have lists, old prescriptions or be able to describe the word of the medication and what it is for, some patients do rely on their significant other to remember the medication for them.

In this case, Royston has suggested that you can speak to his wife for these details. This verbal consent can be used to do the requested task, but do not be tempted to reveal to his wife any further information about Royston, or his eye health, without further consent.

How you choose to approach his wife (should she be there) is down to preference and how you like to run your clinic. You could pop out to ask, request she come in (with Royston's consent) or ask at the end of the test, should you be confident the medication not affect the investigations you are doing (note - if you are dilating - be certain you know the patient's medication prior to using the drops to consider contraindications and drug interactions).

Driving Considerations

Royston's appointment will likely involve a dilation procedure to thoroughly examine his retina and macula. This can cause blurred vision and glare for up to 8 hours, impairing his ability to drive. Therefore, alternative transportation options should be considered. These can include:

1. His wife driving him home.
2. Leaving his car at the location.
3. A neighbour, friend, or relative picking him up.
4. Dropping his car off at home first, then returning via taxi or public transport.

The urgency of the dilation and Royston's current visual standards for driving should also be considered. If his vision is below the required standards, it would be illegal for him to drive. All facts and results should be considered before advising him to inform the DVLA.

Additionally, if a same day referral is required, you will also need to consider how the patient will get there. Eye casualty departments usually prefer the patient to be dilated upon arrival to aid in their triage process.

Whilst these discussions are beyond the scope of the history and symptoms, it is important to have these points in consideration when taking the history as they will affect how you plan the rest of the appointment.

Case #010: Kerry

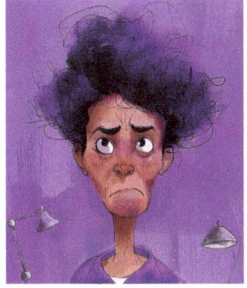

Composition – For the person acting as this patient:

Kerry is a 69-year-old **retired journalist,** who is grumpy and combatant. She is difficult to obtain information from and requires careful wording of questions as to not anger her. She will often reply that she is in a rush, feel like being at the appointment is a waste of time and that answers to all questions "should be written down already". If calmed and reasoned with, she does calm and provide answers in a more relaxed matter.

The red text provides an example of the type of response you should provide to this question
(Smaller text in parenthesis to be used if probed appropriately and/or has managed to build rapport with Kerry)

Please note that this script spans two pages due to the "LOFTSEA" section.

Reason for Visit	"My vision is terrible in the right eye. I've been in the waiting area for ages, surely you should have reviewed my booking notes??"
Last Eye Examination	"I was last seen 6 months ago at Shoes Opticians. Don't your records tell you that?"
Subjective Visual Assessment	"As I told the receptionist! I can't see out of my right eye at all. Get to telling me what is wrong with my eye IMMEDIATELY! I don't have time for all these silly questions!" (If examiner explains why important, say no vision in right eye at all distances. No vision at all – not blurry/not distorted. Just no vision)
Key Symptoms	"NO VISION IN MY RIGHT EYE! WHAT MORE CAN I TELL YOU!?" (If examiner explains why probing as to help with the cause, then say no vision at all in my right eye, no other symptoms are present)
LOFTSEA	
Location	"I'VE TOLD YOU MULTIPLE TIMES IT'S THE RIGHT EYE!"
Onset	"An hour ago. I was told to come straight here"
Frequency	"IT HASN'T IMPROVED SINCE IT HAPPENED! If it had happened before, you'd have thought I could tell you what it was!" (On pressing the importance of question, mention had the top half of vision go for 5 minutes about a month ago but resolved so didn't get it checked out)
Type	"Can't you tell it is significant? I can't see out of my right eye at all!"
Self Treatment	"If I'd have found a way to sort it, don't you think I'd have done that rather than come to you???" (very new and significant symptoms, not able to find anything to help)
Effect on Life	"I'm here, aren't I? I am meant to be going to the theatre with my friends right now and have had to cancel because YOU told me to come in! It had better be worth cancelling for!"
Associated	"Just vision loss. Are we done with this pointless questioning yet?" (No other associated symptoms bar the transient loss - only reveal here if not already mentioned and/or the practitioner pushes for the information)

Ocular History	"I have those variable focal things. Why is this relevant? I can't see!" (Gets on ok otherwise with them. No other hospital eye service/disease)
Family Ocular History	"Mum went blind from macular degeneration. Oh no, you're gonna tell me I have that aren't you? My dad had glaucoma. I'd rather not have that." (Mother macular degeneration, father glaucoma)
General Health	"I am meant to take those statin things for high cholesterol. I bloomin' hate them so don't. Haven't for a few months and I'm not talking to the doctor again, as all they do is nag!" (Only on pressing, reveal that you have diabetes – diet control and diagnosed last year. Underscreening service and no sign of retinopathy)
Medication	"Did I not just say I am meant to be on statins?" (Simvastatin if question the type of statin – note that you are not taking them)
Allergies	"None!"
Family General Health	"Dad died of a stroke. This isn't a sign of a stroke, is it?" (Father had a stroke but no other known health issues in the family)
Hobbies/Interests	"Are you going to get on with finding out what is wrong with me or not?" (Bowls)
Driving Status	"What does this have to do with anything? I don't drive – I never have done either. Waste of time and money!" (Non-driver)
Smoke / Drink	"I came here for my eyes. You aren't going to get all preachy now and tell me off for my lifestyle choices, are you?" (Yes – heavily for 20 years. 25 a day / Non-drinker)
VDU Use	"Only for my emails and correspondence. Had enough when I was working with them every day. Again, how is this relevant to now!?" (Less than an hour a day)
Contact Lenses	"Quit with the sales pitch. I don't want glasses, I don't want contact lenses. I just want you to tell me what on earth is going on with my eye!" (No previous contact lens wear. Not wanting contact lenses)

Reflections on Case #010

Tentative Diagnosis: Right Eye - Central Retinal Artery Occlusion

Kerry has presented with a very sudden onset of total vision loss in one eye, with a history of a transient ischaemic attack in recent history. Whilst Kerry may well be a fiery character, she is most likely highly agitated and terrified about her sudden loss of sight.

There are several points of interest in the case history that should be noted and understood. They may also contribute to Kerry's management plan. Some areas of interest may be duplicate of previous cases. As such, I will highlight case-specific observations that may not have been covered on previous cases.

Medical Emergency

The likely diagnosis in this case is the ocular and medical emergency - central retinal artery occlusion. This is where the there is a blockage of the central retinal artery, preventing blood and oxygen reaching the retina and causing severe damage and eventually death of retinal tissue. This is essentially the patient having a stroke, but with the vessel affected being the eye.

The College of Optometrists* referral guidance is that any complete loss of vision of less that 6 hours duration should be referred to ophthalmology as an emergency. In these cases, every second counts and - should this patient have been triaged correctly, they should have been directed to A&E (with a phonecall from your practice to allow the hospital to know to expect them) and not appeared in your room.

Furthermore, whilst a full script has been included, many questions relating to lifestyle are not relevant to this case. Should you have seen this patient, upon completion of LOFTSEA - checking vision and seeing the fundus would have been my next step, whilst asking further questions about general health and other suspected risk factors whilst they are on the slit lamp - before sending them directly to A&E with a succinct referral letter. In these cases, do not waste time! Find out the key facts and act appropriately!

Quick Tentative Diagnosis

This tentative diagnosis was arrived at based on the complaints of painless, sudden and complete loss of vision with no other presenting symptoms, bar a transient ischaemic attack in her recent history.

There are other causes of sudden vision loss, such as a full retinal detachment, but the case history points us towards a central retinal artery occlusion.

The quicker you can have a working, tentative diagnosis, the quicker you can plan the appointment to ensure the patient gets the care they need. Essentially, Kerry would rather regain her sight in the eye than think your case history was amazing because you found out that she plays bowls and uses her VDU for email!

Aggressive Nature

As mentioned before, Kerry is likely to be acting out of character based on the sudden loss of her vision. People can become defensive or lash out when they are scared. Furthermore, it seems like she was delayed for her appointment - so she may feel annoyed that she wasn't seen on time. Do not take this personally as there are many factors behind a person's behaviour.

That said, you must remain calm and de-escalate the situation (as we have done in case #004 with Desmond). Your safety remains paramount.

With some of the key points of information required to make a tentative diagnosis, the questions may seem pointless to the patient. Try your best to explain the relevance of the questions to her case, whilst remaining empathetic and avoiding becoming defensive.

Thankfully, Kerry's case is unusual - both in presenting pathology and level of difficulty to work with, but having knowledge of how to deal with patients in an emergency will aid in your ability to achieve the best outcome in the most efficient (and safest) way.

Clues in the History

As we've explored in previous cases, the comprehensive information about the patient's LOFTSEA, general health, family health history, and smoking habits significantly contributes to understanding the cause of her vision loss. Her non-adherence to simvastatin treatment, in particular, places her at a heightened risk of a stroke. In her case, she has experienced an ocular stroke. This incident, while alarming, could potentially serve as a crucial early warning sign, helping to prevent a more severe, full-body stroke in the future.

Encourage Compliance

Kerry has been shown not to follow medical advice through not taking her medication and this has resulted in her health being adversely affected. As part of the management plan and referral, encourage her to follow the advice of the medical team that see her to prevent further episodes from occurring.

Additionally, she seemed that she wanted to see her friends instead of coming in - it will be vital to keep this in mind when directing her to the hospital as she may not deem your advice important enough to follow the instructions. If she decides to ignore your direct referral and go to the theatre, then the prognosis of saving vision in the eye is extremely slim - make sure you inform her of this and make note on her record card of the advice provided.

Case #011: Alan

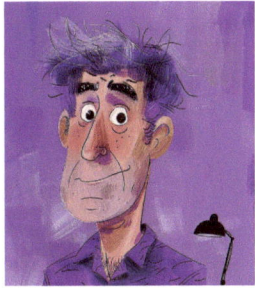

Composition – For the person acting as this patient:

Alan is a contemplative and analytical 58-year-old farmer. He is methodical in his approach to problems and seeks logical explanations for his symptoms. He is cooperative but may appear somewhat perplexed by the changes in his vision.

The green text provides an example of the type of response you should provide to this question
(Smaller text in parenthesis to be used if the practitioner probes appropriately)

Please note that this script spans two pages due to the "LOFTSEA" section.

Reason for Visit	"I'm a bit worried about my left eye - I can't see too far away with it lately, the vision is a bit cloudy, although seem to be able to read with it ok. It's all a bit, well, strange as I don't feel I need glasses anymore!"
Last Eye Examination	"Probably about 5 years ago. Hard to keep up with these appointments, isn't it?"
Subjective Visual Assessment	"Right eye is fine for distance and crystal clear vision, but can't see up close too well. The left eye, as I mentioned is blurry far away, in focus up close but overall poor quality, and kinda yellowy in colour."
Key Symptoms	"Just this change in vision in the left eye really" (On pressing - can reveal gets glare from headlights and sunlight. No flashes, no floaters, no diplopia, no pain, no redness)
LOFTSEA	
Location	"As I was saying, it was my left eye."
Onset	"Probably started, oh approximately 6 months or so ago? It's been gradual but it's becoming more of a problem now."
Frequency	"It's like it all the time. Although sometimes can be worse at times, especially at night or when it is particularly bright!"
Type	"I'd say the symptoms are moderate in nature. I can manage but just confused to what is going on!"
Self Treatment	"I've tried a few things really. Have noticed that it's much better to see all distances if I take my glasses off. Some non-prescription sunglasses and a baseball cap help with the glare and an extra light at night helps me read."
Effect on Life	"I'm liking the fact I don't feel that I need glasses anymore, but am struggling a little when driving at night. It's a nightmare with these oncoming headlights! It's really uncomfortable!"
Associated	"Nothing more than I've said already."

Ocular History	"Told I had the start of cataracts by the last optician, but said they were 'years off'". Other than that, just glasses." (When asked about visits to the eye hospital, say that you have been countless times for foreign body removals)
Family Ocular History	"My mum had cataracts quite early on in life, I think in her early 50s, no other eye diseases I don't think? Well, dad lost an eye on the farm once, but I don't think that counts, right?" (No other eye diseases, no glaucoma)
General Health	"I'm good thanks, fit and active. When you have to be up at 4 am to sort out the farm, it saves having to get a gym membership, that's for sure! That said, haven't been to a doctor's surgery in well over a decade!" (No known general health concerns, no diabetes)
Medication	"My wife makes me take a multivitamin. Does that affect anything?" (None other than the multivitamin)
Allergies	"Rapeseed pollen. Absolute nightmare when this is in season...thankfully none on my farm!"
Family General Health	"My father has arthritis, but otherwise our family are pretty healthy." (No known health issues in the family)
Hobbies/Interests	"Not much time for any of that. But do like to read if I get the time!"
Driving Status	"Of course, car gets me from A to B and of course, I have a few tractors I use to move things between the fields." (Drives without glasses now as finds vision better without them)
Smoke / Drink	"I used to smoke about 20 years ago. Gave it up. Now just enjoy the odd pint of ale at the farm shows." (ex-smoker, 10 a day, smoked for 10 years. Occasional social drinker)
VDU Use	"Rarely. I do plot routes and some of the farm-based software requires some input from me - but I employ a manager to deal with most of the admin and tech stuff!" (Average about 30 minutes a day - desktop)
Contact Lenses	"I don't even think I need glasses now - let alone contact lenses. Not worn them before though as think I'd be a walking infection risk!" (No previous contact lens wear. Not wanting contact lenses)

Reflections on Case #011

Tentative Diagnosis: Left Eye - Nuclear Sclerotic Cataract

Alan has presented with gradual, but significant, visual changes that has changed his refractive status from needing glasses to not needing glasses. He is fairly open and provided a significant amount of information without having to probe too deep with additional questioning. The information he does share is also relevant - making it a different type of encounter than the one we had with Jonathan.

There are several points of interest in the case history that should be noted and understood. They may also contribute to Alan's management plan. Some areas of interest may be duplicate of previous cases. As such, I will highlight case-specific observations that may not have been covered on previous cases.

Myopic Shift

The presentation is one typical of someone who has had a myopic shift caused by progressing nuclear sclerotic cataracts. He states he needed glasses for both distance and near, but has since found he doesn't really need them at all (also commenting at stages that his vision is now worse with them on!).

As the crystalline lens undergoes nuclear sclerosis, the media becomes denser, thus increasing its refractive index and refracting light more. This results in the eye becoming more myopic.

It is likely that Alan was slightly hyperopic prior to the nuclear sclerosis and as such the changes have caused his distance glasses to become overplussed for his needs, blurring the distance. The right eye may very well be close to plano now. The left eye, based on his ability to see up close well with it does indicate that this left eye is now myopic. He has essentially developed monovision - where one eye is set for distance and one eye set for near - and he may be happy to be left this way should a referral not be necessary.

Cataract Risk

There are several parts of the case history that indicate Alan is at risk of developing cataracts, even at a relatively young age.

He is a farmer and spends a significant amount of time outdoors. Therefore he has had a lifetime of ultraviolet exposure, which is a key cause of cataract development. Whilst it is too late to prevent the cataracts developing, discussion on the risk of UV will help prevent further UV damage on his lids and retina. That said, he has already invested in sunglasses - but be sure to educate him on the risk of fake pairs and those not offering 100% UV protection.

He also indicated he used to smoke. Encourage him NOT to resume this hobby (although it is unlikely he will start again now). Remember, smoking is a major risk factor in cataract development.

Finally, he states his mother had cataracts at a young age, hinting that there may be some genetic risk of cataracts developing at his younger age too.

Referral Considerations

Ultimately, the decision to refer will be based on a combination of the patient being diagnosed with a cataract, it being of some visual significance and the patient also wishing to be referred. At present, we have only the case history and no other information, so the following would need to be considered based on what he has told us:

Working age and working: As Alan is working and symptomatic, there is a risk that the cataract could continue to develop and interrupt his ability to work safely and comfortably. Keep this in mind.

Driver: Alan also drives, not only a car but also a tractor. Therefore he needs to have comfortable and clear vision when driving and not experience glare. As he has mentioned glare, this would also have to factor into the decision to refer. Furthermore, you would need to see if he still meets the visual standards for driving when you assess him.

Glare and other symptoms: Whilst Alan is rather enjoying his monovision, he does report symptoms of cloudiness and glare. These symptoms are affecting his life and he is concerned about the symptoms that he has. If you do refer, make sure you include a comment about this on the referral letter.

Other safety considerations: Not asked in this case history, but those presenting with symptomatic cataract should be asked whether or not they have issues with mobility or walking around on uneven ground, as cataracts can affect people in many ways. Check to see if they can read the instructions on their medication, avoid burning themselves when cooking (and other risks that may occur if they are unable to see clearly). Should these be present, make sure they are also recorded on the referral letter and that you suggest ways to help minimise these risks prior to them being seen at the cataract clinic.

Allergies

Alan states that he is allergic to rapeseed pollen, indicating he has some form of hayfever. Whilst it seems like he isn't bothered too badly by it (as it isn't one of his crops), he may encounter an allergic reaction to this whilst working outdoors.

Therefore, you would want to consider assessing the eyes for signs of allergy, discussing ways to relieve him from the allergic response (should he encounter it) and factor in ways that he can mitigate being affected by the pollen in the future (e.g. antihistamines, mast-cell stabilisers and large framed sunglasses), when completing the management part of the eye examination.

Case #012: Michael

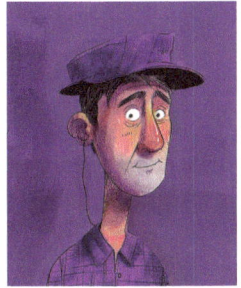

Composition – For the person acting as this patient:

Michael is a 54-year-old, active gardener who enjoys spending time outdoors. He believes he may still have remnants of grass in his eye from a recent gardening mishap, as he sees small, floating shapes that move with his vision. He is somewhat bewildered by these persistent, but painless, symptoms.

The green text provides an example of the type of response you should provide to this question
(Smaller text in parenthesis to be used if the practitioner probes appropriately)

Please note that this script spans two pages due to the "LOFTSEA" section.

Reason for Visit	"I hit myself in the eye a few days ago when pulling some clumps of grass from the verges of my lawn. I think I have grass still in my eye as I can see bits still floating around when I look around!"
Last Eye Examination	"About 3 years ago, something like that"
Subjective Visual Assessment	"Well, all distances seem fine in clarity. But the right eye is bothersome. I can see bits floating around when I look around."
Key Symptoms	"These floating grass bits in my right eye. Big one near my nose!" (Need to press to say shadow/cobweb in vision in superior part of vision towards nose, some flashing in that area too. NO pain, NO diplopia)
LOFTSEA	
Location	"Right eye - mostly towards top part of my vision near my nose"
Onset	"Few days ago now." (on pressing, 2 days ago)
Frequency	"Hmm, actually it has become more noticeable this morning, but it has been constant since it happened"
Type	"Moderate effect on my vision. I've never known grass to do this to my vision before without hurting or irritating the eye"
Self Treatment	"I've tried rinsing the eye a few times with an eye bath, but the grass still appears to be in my vision. I can't seem to wash it out, so figure some must have gotten in through my pupil. I tried rubbing the eye a bit too, but nothing has helped"
Effect on Life	"To be honest, I am baffled to why I can see these things but can't feel them in there. The grass is annoying, but not as annoying as to why I can't work out why I can't feel the grass in my eye"
Associated	"The grass sort of has caused a shadow in my vision. It looks like it flashes in that area sometimes too"

Ocular History	"All pretty good actually. Had a few bits go in my eye throughout the years and they've always been removed ok at the eye hospital" (On pressing, state no known eye diseases)
Family Ocular History	"None that I know of. I'm not even sure what half these conditions are to be honest. How would I be able to find out for you?"
General Health	"Great thanks. Work keeps me active and I've recently been seen by the GP, who tells me I'm very healthy for my age. No diseases, no medication or anything!"
Medication	"As I said, none taken"
Allergies	"I used to get hayfever, but I think I have grown out of it. Other than that, I don't think I am allergic to anything!"
Family General Health	"My father had a heart attack" (No other known health issues in the family)
Hobbies/Interests	"Despite it being my job, I adore gardening."
Driving Status	"I drive my car. And I also ride a bicycle to some of my clients" (On pressing - state that you walked to the appointment today)
Smoke / Drink	"I don't smoke. I do enjoy a beer upon completion of a big job though!"
VDU Use	"A couple of hours a week here and there. Mainly to check for emails and designs from my clients. Occasionally play Tetris on my phone on my break, but that is it."
Contact Lenses	"Never needed a pair of glasses more than the ready readers off the peg. Not sure why I'd want contact lenses - especially as I can't even get this grass out of my eye!"

Reflections on Case #012

Tentative Diagnosis: Right Eye - Suspect Retinal Tear/Detachment

Michael has come in as a patient who appears confused by his symptoms. His eye condition is more serious than what his initial complaints might suggest. It is crucial not to rely solely on a patient's self-diagnosis. Instead, we should always conduct a thorough investigation of the symptoms presented to avoid overlooking any key findings. Although this case is fictional, it's based on a real case I encountered during my hospital placement in the pre-registration period - which demonstrates that these types of encounters do exist!

There are several points of interest in the case history that should be noted and understood. They may also contribute to Michael's management plan. Some areas of interest may be duplicate of previous cases. As such, I will highlight case-specific observations that may not have been covered on previous cases.

Red Herring?

Michael is presenting with symptoms that, from taking his words literally, indicate he has a foreign body (or foreign bodies!) in his eye. From his perspective, he hit his eye with some garden material that he believes he can see floating in his eyes. Without probing further, a practitioner may be temped to do an anterior eye assessment only and not detect what the true cause is.

Essentially, he is explaining he has a sudden onset of floaters in his vision that came on directly after blunt trauma to the eye, with the presence of some flashing lights and a shadow in his vision - the hallmark set of symptoms that occur when there is a retinal tear or detachment. Ultimately, in the case this was based on, the patient did have a substantial tear on their retina.

Remember, just because a patient thinks it is something, don't be negligent and assume they must be correct - investigate further and explore differential diagnoses too! It's not to say the patient is always wrong (as quite often they are right!) but to make sure you use your expertise to rule out other serious causes of their symptoms.

Check it Makes Sense

Foreign bodies often cause significant ocular discomfort, redness and watering of the eyes, with significant foreign bodies causing photophobia (sensitivity to light). Michael doesn't have these symptoms - just the appearance of floating bits in his eye.

Therefore, your thoughts of a foreign body being the reason for the symptoms should be replaced with other tentative diagnoses - especially as removing the context of it being "grass in the eye", this is a presentation of flashes and floaters.

Always take the time to consider if the symptoms make sense to the presentation - if they don't probe further and perform additional investigations.

Eye Protection

Whilst it may be a little too late to protect his eyes from the trauma caused in this case, it would be advisable that you discuss eye protection with him.

He enjoys being in the garden and, with his work, he is likely to encounter many threats to his eyes. Rose thorns, twigs, bamboo canes, mud, dirt, seeds - all are common sources of ocular threat and as such, you should discuss this with him as to prevent eye injuries in the future.

This discussion on eye protection should also occur even if he is presenting as a routine patient - not only have we identified that the garden is a source of ocular injury, but his ocular history also indicates his eyes have had many encounters with foreign bodies - prompting you to have this discussion.

Patient Observation

Michael has stated he works outdoors and enjoys time outdoors. One of the biggest threat to his eyes in the ultraviolet light from the sun. Looking at Michael, you can observe he has evidence of sunburn - especially on his nose.

It would be prudent to inform him the risk of ultraviolet light has on his health - and encourage ultraviolet blocking eyewear (perhaps consider this with safety goggles also) to minimise damage to his eyes; lowering the risk for subsequent cataracts and macular degeneration.

The sunburn can also be of concern as this could lead to skin cancers, often affecting the lids and periorbital areas. As such discussing eye protection, alongside other general healthcare tips about looking after his health in the sun would be something to consider from this presentation.

Keep it Relevant

Again, this presentation is an ocular emergency and time is a factor. This presentation is not a routine eye examination and Michael will be more likely to recommend your services if you are to the point, identify what the cause of his symptoms are and refer appropriately than consider how thorough your case history is because you went on to ask about his smoking and drinking status, how often he uses a computer and what he likes to do in his spare time.

Whilst this information is important in understanding Michael, in this presentation, ideally you want to be able to diagnose the cause and manage appropriately - so if you do need to ask these questions, do so when investigating (there is nothing stopping you asking case history questions whilst you are performing examinations or writing/typing up your notes).

Case #013: Dilys

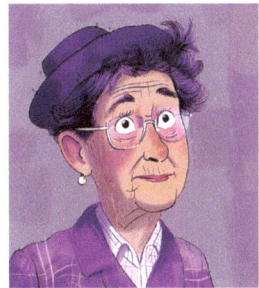

Composition – For the person acting as this patient:

Dilys is a very shy and reserved 95-year-old **retired librarian**. She speaks softly and may need gentle encouragement to share her concerns. She has a limited understanding of eye-related terminology and expresses her symptoms in simple terms.

Reveal only bold & purple text when asked **but when probed further, add detail from non-bold text**

Please note that this script spans two pages due to the "LOFTSEA" section.

Reason for Visit	"My vision has changed. I'm not sure how to describe it"
Last Eye Examination	"It's been so long, I'm not entirely sure. Maybe 10 years?"
Subjective Visual Assessment	"Perhaps it's a little more difficult to see far away. I also have to hold things much closer than I used to see them"
Key Symptoms	"Just feel I need new glasses" (No red flag symptoms upon questioning)
LOFTSEA	
Location	"Both of my eyes"
Onset	"Oh goodness, it must be about 2-3 years ago that I started to notice it but more obvious recently"
Frequency	"All the time" (On pressing, mention more obvious at night or lower light conditions)
Type	"Hmm, it is just haziness and blurriness of my vision in both eyes"
Self Treatment	"I've taken my glasses off for reading now. I also find a lamp helps when I am needing to read things" (If presses further, mention that need sunglasses when out and about because of the glare that is experienced in brighter conditions)
Effect on Life	"It's annoying to have to take my glasses off to read. And the brightness when I'm out and about is tough!" (On pressing, mention it is the reason that you stopped driving)
Associated	"Everything is dim to see and it is harder to read newspapers" (If presses further, mention the issues you have with glare).

Ocular History	"None that I am aware of. Just needed glasses" (If asked about cataracts, state that the last optician you saw said you had some cataracts that she wanted to monitor, but haven't thought more of it)
Family Ocular History	"None that I know of" (No known cataracts or glaucoma)
General Health	"They said that I am fairly good for my age. I take a pill for my blood pressure. And they tell me to take a statin" (On direct asking about diabetes, state that you are pre-diabetic)
Medication	"A white one for my blood pressure. And that statin" (On pressing for a name, mimic searching for a repeat prescription and read off: bendroflumethiazide, atenolol, alendronic acid, atorvastatin, rivaroxaban and senna)
Allergies	"Antibiotics of some sort" (On pressing - penicillin. Only had reaction as child, caused a minor rash)
Family General Health	"My father had a heart attack, mum died of old age" (No other known health issues in the family, no diabetes)
Hobbies/Interests	"Cross-stitch, knitting. Crosswords too"
Driving Status	"I don't drive anymore. I gave that up because I didn't feel confident with my vision"
Smoke / Drink	"I have never smoked. My late husband smoked and I could never get used to the smell. I don't drink either"
VDU Use	"If you count the television, I watch quite a bit. My daughter bought me a phone but I don't really know how to work it. I dare not go near a computer"
Contact Lenses	"Do you think I need them for my eye problem?" (Never used them, not interested)

Reflections on Case #013

Tentative Diagnosis: Bilateral Cataracts - Likely Nuclear Sclerotic / Mixed

Dilys has presented after a long absence from the care of an optometrist and has noticed gradual, but significant changes to her vision. Her symptoms indicate a myopic shift - making distance vision more difficult, as well as causing her to have to hold things much closer to read. The subtle hints of glare, coupled with reduced contrast would suggest this is caused by media opacities - most likely nuclear sclerotic cataracts with a mix of other cataract types.

There are several points of interest in the case history that should be noted and understood. They may also contribute to Dilys' management plan. Some areas of interest may be duplicate of previous cases. As such, I will highlight case-specific observations that may not have been covered on previous cases.

Probe Further

Dilys does provide some information but she is still relatively reserved compared to other patients that we have encountered in this book. Some of her responses only tell half the story and require you to take extra time to investigate the answers further.

Missed History?

When inquiring about her overall health, she mentions that she's only on two medications. However, it's important to note that when asked directly about a potential diabetes diagnosis, she discloses that she is pre-diabetic. This highlights the importance of asking specific questions related to common medical conditions such as diabetes, hypertension, glaucoma, and macular degeneration. Patients often omit these conditions when asked open-ended questions about their health history.

Furthermore, it could have been easy to suggest that this voluntary offering of medication provides the complete list of her medication and underlying health issues. If you probed further, she does retrieve a medication list with other medication. This medication does indicate she has other undisclosed health complaints that may be useful to know about (notably the rivaroxaban being a blood thinner and alendronic acid used in osteoporosis).

Penicillin Allergies

Allergies can range in severity from causing mild discomfort to triggering life-threatening anaphylaxis. It's crucial to identify the actual allergen and understand its impact on the patient.

In the past, penicillin was administered in high doses, which led to adverse reactions in many patients, resulting in it being recorded as an allergen. However, the dosages used today are significantly lower. Understanding how the drug affected the patient can provide secondary care providers with valuable insights and treatment options for potential infections.

Case #014: Noah

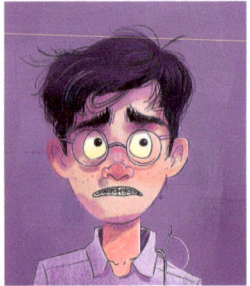

Composition – For the person acting as this patient:

Noah is a 17-year-old sixth form student. He has been booked in by his mum, who is concerned about his complaints of blurry vision, especially at the end of the day. Noah is not impressed to be here as he is missing out on hanging out with his friends at the local football game.

The red text provides an example of the type of response you should provide to this question
(Smaller text in parenthesis to be used if probed appropriately and/or has managed to build rapport with Noah)

Please note that this script spans two pages due to the "LOFTSEA" section.

Reason for Visit	"Mum told me to come. Aren't you supposed to know that?"
Last Eye Examination	"Couple of months? You gave me these glasses, remember?"
Subjective Visual Assessment	"Glasses are ok, right? But sometimes my vision goes a bit weird. Like distance and up close can be blurry. But not all the time"
Key Symptoms	"Blurry every now and again. Sometimes see two of everything when it happens and makes my head hurt" (Eyestrain type symptoms. No flashes, no floaters, no photophobia)
LOFTSEA	
Location	"Both of my eyes. Aches and pains around my eyes."
Onset	"Dunno really. Few weeks?"
Frequency	"Most days. Happens at end of the day or when I've been gaming or doing homework" (if pressed, only when gaming on phone/table/doing homework on laptop)
Type	"Just this blurring and eyestrain thing"
Self Treatment	"It's easier if I work on a proper computer or if I game on the TV in the lounge, but mum doesn't let me play on the downstairs TV that often" (If pressed, say that taking a break also makes it go away after 30 mins)
Effect on Life	"Frustrating. I can't do anything when it happens. It makes me miserable. I reckon it is these glasses you gave me!"
Associated	"It makes me tired and irritable!"

Ocular History	"These glasses. You said I was short-sighted" (No other ocular history)
Family Ocular History	"Mum and dad wear glasses" (No known cataracts or glaucoma, no other eye diseases)
General Health	"I'm alright. I play football every now and again. Why do you wanna know?" (No health issues, no diabetes, no hypertension)
Medication	"Just one for hayfever" (On pressing for a name - say "ask me mum, she's outside" - Loratadine"
Allergies	"Hayfever" (On pressing - penicillin. Only had reaction as child, caused a minor rash)
Family General Health	"Nan had diabetes, nothing else that I know of" (No other known health issues in the family)
Hobbies/Interests	"Support Advocate United - was meant to be going to their game, but mum booked this in for me. Call of Duty, Fortnite and all those sorts of games. I play them all night!"
Driving Status	"Going to learn this year, hopefully!"
Smoke / Drink	"Umm, I'm too young to drink and smoke. Why do you ask?"
VDU Use	"What's a VDU?" (when reworded about screen use - say high use. 3 hours laptop for homework, then 3-5 hours minimum gaming. Prefers handheld console. Uses mobile phone all day too)
Contact Lenses	"I want them. Mum says they are too expensive for me at the moment" (Interested, but may not be able to afford them)

Reflections on Case #014

Tentative Diagnosis: Refractive / Accommodative Spasm

Noah is here because his mum has made him present for an appointment. Thankfully he is relatively open, if not a little put out for being here, so only moderate probing for more information is needed. Given the symptoms and history, the issue he is experiencing is likely aesthenopia (eyestrain and headaches) caused either by an incorrect refractive error - or more likely, accommodative spasm.

There are several points of interest in the case history that should be noted and understood. They may also contribute to Noah's management plan. Some areas of interest may be duplicate of previous cases. As such, I will highlight case-specific observations that may not have been covered on previous cases.

Intermittent and Temporary Blurring

Noah informs us that his symptoms come and go and only last a short amount of time, with the primary symptom being blurring of vision. This is where the LOFTSEA questions come in particularly useful, as it will attempt to reveal to us what triggers these symptoms and what effect they are having on him.

This deeper dive reveals that the symptoms tend to come on later in the day and are strongly related to prolonged near tasks, such as homework and videogames. Furthermore, the symptoms tend to resolve shortly after relaxing the eyes. This predominantly points to an accommodative issue (such as accommodative spasm), but could also point the his prescription being overminused - forcing him to accommodate more than he needs to. Therefore your test should plan to assess refraction, binocular vision and accommodative functions.

Screen Use

As we have mentioned above, the near demands for Noah are high. Therefore it would be advisable to discuss screen use with him - aiming to reduce the amount of time he uses a screen, reminding him to take regular breaks and also consider increasing the working distance he is using the screen at also (if you recall, he finds using the TV in the lounge easier than using his tablet or laptop).

Managing the screen use will likely be the main management in this case, unless any other findings during the eye examination reveal otherwise.

Contact Lenses

Noah is interested in contact lens use, but has been told they are too expensive by his mum. It may be worth, if Noah consents, you discussing contact lenses with his mum, providing prices and details as this may be a worthwhile option for both Noah and the practice.   There are many contact lenses available now and with a wide range of prices. You may be surprised that patients do not know this and just the act of educating the patient may be enough to let them decide to give them a try.

Myopia Control

The vision problems Noah is experiencing could potentially be linked to the use of myopia control lenses in his glasses. The case history doesn't clarify whether these lenses are in his current pair, although previous records could provide this information. However, it's important to note that these symptoms wouldn't fluctuate throughout the day but would likely remain constant in their severity.

If Noah isn't currently using myopia control lenses, it might be beneficial to consider them when recommending new glasses, especially if his prescription has changed. Even though the main issue at hand isn't related to the progression of myopia, it doesn't mean that managing his myopia isn't important.

Moreover, given the significant amount of time Noah spends in front of a screen, it's crucial to discuss the risk of myopia progression. He should be advised to take regular breaks, increase the distance between him and his screens, and ensure he spends ample time outdoors.

"What's a VDU"

Noah's innocent reply to our question on VDU usage has gently reminded us of the importance of carefully choosing our words when communicating with our patients. It's crucial to avoid using technical terms and acronyms when discussing or explaining matters to our patients to prevent any confusion.

Using jargon can create barriers to understanding and may make patients feel alienated or overwhelmed. It's important to remember that while these terms are familiar to us as healthcare professionals, they can be confusing and intimidating to those without a medical background.

Additionally, using clear and simple language can help build trust between healthcare providers and patients. When patients understand what's being said, they're more likely to feel comfortable and engaged in their care. This can lead to better patient satisfaction, improved adherence to treatment plans, and ultimately, better health outcomes.

Driving Status

Noah has informed us that he is planning to learn to drive this year. Therefore it is imperative to make sure that he is meeting the visual requirements required for driving, as well as ensuring his symptoms are controlled. It is vital to inform him whether or not he will need to wear his glasses to drive - so factor this into any management plan that you build on completion of the appointment.

Cycloplegic Examination

In cases where accommodative issues may be affecting the overall refraction, you may wish to consider a cycloplegic examination. If this is the case, consider the order of tests you are going to perform, whether it is indicated to do urgently (as you can defer/rebook depending on patient need and clinical demands) and other aspects you may uncover during the examination.

Case #015: Laura

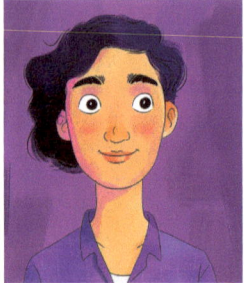

Composition – For the person acting as this patient:

Laura is a 34-year-old financial advisor who is experiencing visual disturbances that she describes as 'flickering lights' and 'zigzag patterns' in her vision. She is articulate and provides a clear description of her symptoms, which she notes are affecting her ability to work. She is concerned but calm, seeking an explanation for these episodes.

The green text provides an example of the type of response you should provide to this question
Please note that this script spans two pages due to the "LOFTSEA" section.

Reason for Visit	"Over the last 6 months I've been experiencing 20-minute episodes of zig zags in my vision.. They often come before a headache. Spoke to the GP and he recommended an eye exam."
Last Eye Examination	"About a year ago"
Subjective Visual Assessment	"Vision is fine - other than when these zig-zags appear and then everything is hard to see for about 20 minutes at all distances"
Key Symptoms	"Zig-zag like flashes in my vision that cause a nasty headache afterwards. Nothing else. No floaty bits or doubling of vision"
LOFTSEA	
Location	"Both of my eyes see it, but think more on the right hand side."
Onset	"Started at the same time I qualified. So about 6 months"
Frequency	"A couple of times a week. Often towards the end of a particularly busy day or when I've dealt with stressful clients"
Type	"It can be significant - obscuring my vision for about 20 minutes. Then sometimes the headache after can be very severe!"
Self Treatment	"I've found they don't happen on days where I am not stressed. If I'm home, I lie down in a dark room and that helps to prevent the headache. Painkillers can help a little"
Effect on Life	"It can be significant. I can't see to work when the zig zags appear and then can't focus with the subsequent headache!"
Associated	"Bar the headache after, I can feel quite nauseous, cold and shaky. It isn't pleasant. Lights and sounds can feel more intense too!"

Ocular History	"I sometimes wear the reading glasses you prescribed last time for near work. They don't make much difference. I was referred a few years back for a birthmark on the retina of my right eye, but discharged as a congenital mark that they weren't worried about"
Family Ocular History	"Mum has glaucoma and is treated with drops and the same for my older brother. Dad has the start of cataracts."
General Health	"They are watching me for high blood pressure, they think that has been caused by stress. I also have terrible circulation in my hands and feet. I also have been told I have early type 2 diabetes, so am awaiting the start of treatment. If that wasn't enough I am also under a sleep clinic as my partner notices I snore VERY loudly and occasionally stop breathing at night! I seem to have it all!" (if asked, not pregnant or breastfeeding)
Medication	"Ramipril for the blood pressure. Nothing else yet but they said they are likely to put me on metformin very soon"
Allergies	"Guinea pig dander. I love the little critters but holding them makes me come out in a rash!"
Family General Health	"Both parents and a brother have type 2 diabetes. Seems its a family based thing. Dad had a stroke 3 years ago"
Hobbies/Interests	"Yoga is a big interest for me as it really does lessen the stress I feel at work. Occasionally I like to hit the beach and paint the landscape, but I've not had the time as of late!"
Driving Status	"I drive a car, mainly for work"
Smoke / Drink	"I smoked socially as a teenager, but stopped by age 20. I have the occasional glass of wine"
VDU Use	"All day. Every day. If it isn't checking emails and assessing the market updates, it is planning reports and catching up with clients via video conferences. 9-10 hours a day 5 days a week. Then the odd movie on my laptop at weekends"
Contact Lenses	"I don't even get on too well with the glasses you prescribed, so I don't think I need contact lenses!"

Reflections on Case #015

Tentative Diagnosis: Classic Migraine

Laura is a lovely patient to take a history from as she is comprehensive in her symptoms, conveys the information directly and provides additional context, without waffling. You may have noticed that there were no additional texts to the script, meaning she provided enough information per question that you could use for each section and for you to make a tentative diagnosis. Keep in mind, whilst some patients like this provide a lot of information, it is still important to delve deeper should any areas seem unexplained or require further explanation.

There are several points of interest in the case history that should be noted and understood. They may also contribute to Laura's management plan. Some areas of interest may be duplicate of previous cases. As such, I will highlight case-specific observations that may not have been covered on previous cases.

Zig-Zags and Flashes

Laura is worried about seeing flashing zig-zags in her vision, which then turn into a big headache. This is a common symptom of classic migraines.

When a migraine happens, it's like an "electrical storm" moving across the brain. If it moves over the parts of the brain used for seeing, it can make the person see flashing lights or zig-zags. These usually happen 20 minutes before the headache starts, but sometimes they can happen without a headache at all.

It's important to note that these flashes are very different from the ones a person might see if they have a tear or detachment in their retina. However, any kind of flashes should be taken seriously to rule out other serious causes.

Pigmented Lesion

Laura has mentioned that she has a "birthmark" on her right eye. She has been told that it's not harmful, so she has been discharged from further medical care for it.

Given this information, it's crucial to make sure you look for, evaluate, and document that you have seen this mark during your examination. You should be confident enough to confirm its benign nature at the end of the appointment.

Not recording it in the medical records after being informed about it could suggest that you didn't notice it. This could lead to problems if there are any issues with the mark in the future. For instance, questions could arise such as: Did you overlook it during the examination? Or did you fail to record its existence?

To avoid such situations, it's always best to document all findings, even if they are considered benign. This ensures that all information is available for future reference and can help in tracking any changes over time.

Migraines

An overarching theme of Laura's case history is her battle with stress. Stress is highly prevalent among professionals, and undoubtedly, during your studies and clinical career, you'll encounter it as well.

Stress can act as a trigger for migraines, which might explain why Laura experiences them so frequently. This stress could be compounded by the significant amount of time she spends on her computer—partly contributing to her stress and also causing prolonged near-focus, leading to eyestrain and subsequently contributing to her migraines.

Recommending Laura keep a migraine diary—a record of her activities, emotions, and dietary choices leading up to each migraine. Identifying triggers can help her avoid further migraines. Discussing common triggers, such as the "five C's of migraines" (cheese, chocolate, claret (red wines), caffeine, and citrus fruits), may also help her pinpoint the causes. Additionally managing her stress and screen use will also likely help minimise the frequency that she encounters them.

If all examination ocular findings are normal, consider advising Laura to consult her GP. Migraines may have other underlying causes that need investigation. The GP can also prescribe tablets to prevent or reduce migraines, effectively assisting Laura.

Risk Factors

Whilst Laura is presenting with symptoms of a migraine, she also reveals significant risk factors for developing an open angle glaucoma. These risk factors are:

- Strong family history of glaucoma
- Hypertension
- Diabetes
- Migraine
- Raynaud's phenomenon/poor circulation
- Sleep Apnea
- History of smoking

All of these are risk factors for glaucoma, thus you would need to consider performing a glaucoma work-up as part of the appointment to rule out the presence of glaucoma.

Closing Notes on Case Study Selection 2

This section covered patients presenting with visual concerns; ranging from emerging presbyopia to wet macular degeneration. These patients will make a significant proportion of the appointments that you see, albeit often skewed towards refractive-based origins.

Whilst these cases will be managed differently to a routine appointment, these case histories are vital to help establish a differential diagnosis of their presenting complaints. Performing practice sessions with these case notes will allow you to understand where you need to focus your questions to keep the appointment relevant for that patient.

Reason for Visit Patients presenting with concerns can sometimes feel overwhelming, but keep in mind that these are the issues that they want you to solve. If they are saying the vision is cloudy in the right eye – then you will be looking at investigating the cause of cloudy vision in that right eye. Whilst a thorough history will still be important, it will be a source of your attention, weighting the questioning towards finding the cause of that presenting history.

Family Clues Many of these patients had health and family history issues that would help to shed light on the cause of their presenting concerns. Kerry, who smoked, drank a lot of alcohol, had hypertension and high cholesterol had all the health risk factors of a stroke (of which her father also suffered) and the underlying cause of her symptoms was an ophthalmic transient ischaemic attack. Don't just go through the motions when asking the case history. Build up that patient's visual status, risk profile and their presenting needs to ensure you are helping them at every level.

Glasses Talk Many of the conditions here didn't focus too much on refractive concerns (bar the presbyopia cases). It is important to consider refractive causes in each case, but if a patient is referring to transient vision loss, flashes, floaters or distortion – it is highly unlikely that their spectacles are the cause. Therefore, if you suspect pathology – orientate the questions around finding the cause rather than gearing the conversation about what they could improve in their current eyewear. However, in cases where the cause of their visual concern is likely refractive – then do consider spending the time discussing how to improve that with new eyewear.

Contact Lens Chat

As described in the glasses talk section, you aren't going to want to steer a discussion about trying contact lenses in a patient that has symptoms highly suggestive of an imminent referral. Be adaptable to what you focus on and what you may only wish to touch upon (or in some cases, neglect to discuss). In ophthalmic emergencies, time is of the essence, and it is not in anyone's interest to be discussing the merits of types of presbyopia correction contact lenses can solve whilst said patient's retina is falling off!

That said, if the cause is likely contact lens related (they've put too many in, or it's vision loss due to contact lens abuse!) then do investigate with further questions about their contact lenses and their habits.

Types of Patient and Emotions

Again, we covered a range of patients with different demeanours during this section. It is always important to keep in mind that those experiencing a visual concern will be anxious about what you will find. This anxiety may be displayed as quietness, aggression or, in some cases, nonchalance. Read your patient throughout and act accordingly. Always be empathetic and genuine, as this will aid rapport building, obtaining further information from them whilst aiding your investigations.

In a nutshell, this section delved into patients showing up with visual worries, from presbyopia creeping in to ophthalmic strokes. These patients will fill a good chunk of your appointments, though they tend to lean toward refractive issues. So, when you're chatting with them, focus on what's bothering them—whether it's cloudy vision or a need for new specs. And remember, if their retina's falling off, maybe save the contact lens sales pitch for a future appointment!

Case Study Selection 3
Ocular Pain and Discomfort

This chapter delves into the clinical encounters with patients experiencing eye pain or discomfort. While such cases may not constitute a significant portion of your daily clinic schedule, they are nonetheless a recurring scenario, presenting themselves several times throughout the week. It's essential for eye care professionals to be well-versed in handling these conditions, despite their relative infrequency.

The investigation of eye pain and discomfort presents a complex challenge for optometrists, primarily due to the subjective nature of pain. What one patient may describe as a mild irritation could be debilitating pain for another. This subjectivity therefore requires a nuanced approach to diagnosis and treatment. Pain's manifestation can range from an acute, sudden onset to a chronic, lingering condition. It may vary in intensity throughout the day and show different responses to various treatment modalities.

As you progress through these patient case scenarios, the critical role of strategic questioning becomes clear. You will need to employ a combination of open-ended and closed questions to allow you to gather comprehensive information about the patient's presenting needs. In certain instances, it may be necessary to delve deeper with additional queries to uncover the root cause of the discomfort. This methodical approach is key in developing a solid working diagnosis to formulate an effective assessment of the patient to reach the core of the presenting complaint.

It's important to recognise that examining patients who are experiencing severe eye pain can be particularly challenging for several reasons. These individuals may exhibit signs of fatigue, which can be attributed to the emotional toll of enduring intense pain. In some cases, the discomfort may escalate to a point where it provokes irritability or aggression. Additionally, the severity of the pain might impede standard assessment procedures, as patients could struggle to keep their eyes open for examination. It's crucial to bear in mind that as a healthcare professional, you must adhere to your certified scope of practice and refrain from performing any procedures for which you lack proper training and insurance for. Therefore, a thorough case history that can lead to a tentative diagnosis is essential should you need to urgently refer this patient on to another professional.

Please remember that all of the following cases are fictional patients, but representing real-world presentations. Any similarities to people, real or fictional, is purely co-incidental.

Case #016: Morgan

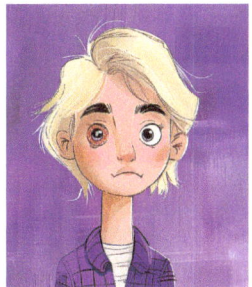

Composition – For the person acting as this patient:

Morgan is a 20-year-old, active **English literature student** who enjoys swimming. She presents with a red and painful eye that has occurred after a swimming session. She is very exhausted from the pain and it is clear the discomfort has drained her completely.

Reveal only bold & purple text when asked **but when probed further, add detail from non-bold text**
Please note that this script spans two pages due to the "LOFTSEA" section.

Reason for Visit	"My right eye is really red and painful. I just need it to stop"
Last Eye Examination	"About a year ago"
Subjective Visual Assessment	"Vision is not good in my right eye. My left eye is fine with my contact lenses in"
Key Symptoms	"Pain. So painful. And red" (Painful red eye, light sensitive, watery. No flashes, no floaters nor diplopia)
LOFTSEA	
Location	"Right eye"
Onset	"3 am this morning" (Pain caused me to wake up)
Frequency	"Constantly there, it is relentless"
Type	"The pain is horrendous. I've never felt pain like it"
Self Treatment	"I took my contact lenses out, but the pain only got worse" (Tried an ocular lubricant and eye bath to see if it washed any debris in my eye away, but it made no difference)
Effect on Life	"The pain is so bad that I cannot do anything. I don't even want to be here. Just make the pain stop"
Associated	"There appears to be a white patch on my eye. It thought it was part of the contact lens, but it came out complete"

Ocular History	"I am short-sighted, I wear contact lenses. I've never had anything in the eye like this before! I hate glasses, they're so heavy!" (No hospital visits, no eye disease. If asked if wore the contact lenses swimming, say that you did and that you always do without problem)
Family Ocular History	"Mum and dad wear glasses" (No known eye diseases)
General Health	"My health is fine" (No health complaints, no diabetes, no hypertension, not pregnant/breastfeeding)
Medication	"Just the pill"
Allergies	"None"
Family General Health	"They're ok" (Mum has diabetes, dad has asthma)
Hobbies/Interests	"Swimming" (Water polo, diving)
Driving Status	"I drive" (car only, wears contact lenses when driving)
Smoke / Drink	"No to both"
VDU Use	"Please help me with this pain" (4 hours a day, prefers to read from a book than a screen, but needs to write essays for university course)
Contact Lenses	"Yes. I've worn them for 2 years"
Further CL Details	**ONLY GIVE THE BELOW INFORMATION WHEN ASKED**
Lens Type	"The Advocate Breathe 1-Day"
Age of Current Lenses	"About 3 weeks old"
Average Wear Time	"All day every day"
Solutions Used	"No solutions - I bin them when I take them out"
Swimming in Lenses?	"Yes, you can't expect me to wear glasses in the pool!"
Showering in Lenses?	"Yes"
Sleeping in Lenses?	"Yes"

Reflections on Case #016

Tentative Diagnosis: Right Eye Microbial Keratitis - Suspect Acanthamoeba Keratitis

Morgan is clearly in pain at this appointment, the discomfort that she is experiencing has severely drained her and she is not able to engage very well. She will answer questions but it takes a lot of effort from both sides to transmit the answers.

There are several points of interest in the case history that should be noted and understood. They may also contribute to Morgan's management plan. Some areas of interest may be duplicate of previous cases. As such, I will highlight case-specific observations that may not have been covered on previous cases.

Contact Lens Misuse

Morgan's situation arises from improper use of her contact lenses, revealing several unsafe practices in her case history (had the right questions been asked!).

Wearing contact lenses for extended periods or while sleeping can deprive the cornea of oxygen, potentially leading to ulceration and subsequent infection. Given the severity of her symptoms and her observation of a large lesion on the front of her eye, it strongly suggests an ulcer, likely infected due to the intense pain.

Our primary concern in Morgan's case revolves around water exposure while wearing lenses. Most water sources harbour various microbes, but our greatest worry is acanthamoeba—a tiny, single-celled protozoan capable of causing serious eye damage. Activities like swimming, showering, or allowing contact lenses to come into contact with water significantly elevate the risk of developing this condition.

Management necessitates an emergency referral to ophthalmology. If you suspect acanthamoeba keratitis, explicitly state it in the referral so that the patient can undergo appropriate investigation and treatment. Additionally, if Morgan intends to resume contact lens wear in the future, emphasise strict education on safe contact lens practices.

I strongly recommend discussing contact lens compliance with all of your contact lens patients. Assess their ability to wear lenses safely and take the opportunity to address and correct risky behaviors. Many patients remain unaware of the risks associated with contact lens misuse, and it's unclear whether these conversations are actually occurring at fitting appointments (they should be!) or if patients simply believe the rules don't apply to them. Either way, make sure that you are confident that the patient is aware of the risks and what to do if they encounter an issue when they are wearing contact lenses.

Contact Lens Questions

Even during primary care appointments, it's essential to address contact lens use. Although the focus may not be on contact lens aftercare, discussing lenses with your patient remains relevant.

While a significant, painful, and red eye can occur without contact lens wear, certain cases are linked to lens use. Asking about their contact lens habits helps narrow down potential causes. If the patient reports not wearing lenses, it rules out conditions associated with contact lens use.

Additional questions related to contact lens wear play a crucial role. Digging deeper into the specifics can provide valuable insights. For instance, understanding the modality of lens wear (daily, extended, or occasional), the average wear time, the type of lenses used, and their overall contact lens habits can further hone in on the underlying issue. Some causes may be linked to poor compliance with lens wear, while others could result from deposits accumulating on the lenses. Additionally, an ill-fitting lens might contribute to the symptoms. These further inquiries serve as useful pointers in identifying the cause and guiding appropriate management

Pain

Acanthamoeba keratitis is among the most excruciating conditions a person can experience. When a patient presents with this condition, assessing them becomes exceptionally challenging.

As an eye care professional, empathy is crucial. However, some assessments may inadvertently worsen their symptoms. For instance:

- **Bright Lights**: Using the slit lamp or ophthalmoscope can intensify their pain and photophobia.

- **Eye Examination**: Touching their eyelids to open their eyes for corneal examination poses difficulties.

In cases requiring immediate referral, prioritise assembling a tentative diagnosis and documenting relevant details for your ophthalmology colleagues. Avoid unnecessary tests that contribute little clinical value (e.g. binocular vision or color vision testing just for the purpose of completing their record card).

Remember that pain alters behavior. Morgan, typically upbeat and chatty, now withdraws due to intense pain. Other patients might become agitated or aggressive. Strive to extract essential information using minimal tests, so you can get them on their journey to relief as soon as you can.

Case #017: Jack

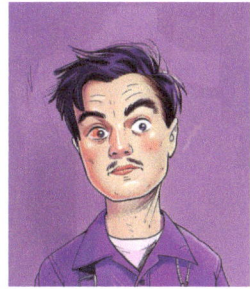

Composition – For the person acting as this patient:

Jack is a 32-year-old car mechanic who is accustomed to hands-on work. He presents with discomfort in his right eye, suspecting that a small piece of metal or debris has entered it while working. He is straightforward and practical, seeking a quick and effective solution to his problem.

Reveal only bold & purple text when asked **but when probed further, add detail from non-bold text**
Please note that this script spans two pages due to the "LOFTSEA" section.

Reason for Visit	"I think I got something in my eye" (Right eye, was working under a car and felt something go in)
Last Eye Examination	"Think I had one when I was a young kid. I can see just fine so never have them checked"
Subjective Visual Assessment	"My right eye is a little blurry, but think it is because it is watering a lot from there being something in it"
Key Symptoms	"Feels like there is something in the eye. A bit uncomfortable and red" (Watery eye, slightly light sensitive. No flashes, no floaters, no diplopia)
LOFTSEA	
Location	"Right eye"
Onset	"Suddenly happened about 3 hours ago, I was working under a car"
Frequency	"Constant sensation since the bit fell in. Reckon a bit of metal?"
Type	"Quite uncomfortable if I am honest. Nearly painful, especially in this bright room"
Self Treatment	"Rinsed the eye with our work's eye bath thing, still sore" (Work mate checked and could see something there after rinsing and said to get it checked)
Effect on Life	"I'm just worried something is stuck there to be honest. Its uncomfortable and I can't work with it like it is!"
Associated	"Wateriness. No gunk like it is infected though. Can be sensitive with lights!"

Ocular History	"You're the first person I remember ever seeing for my eyes if I'm honest" (No known eye disease, no ophthalmology visits, no glasses)
Family Ocular History	"My dad reads with glasses that's it. Didn't even know you could get eye diseases if I am honest" (No known eye diseases)
General Health	"My health is fine" (No health complaints, no diabetes, no hypertension etc)
Medication	"Don't take nothing"
Allergies	"None"
Family General Health	"They're ok" (Mum has breast cancer, dad has diabetes)
Hobbies/Interests	"Football. Quite like having a kick about with the lads after work on a Friday. Got a season ticket to Advocate United too!"
Driving Status	" I love driving. Have a car but also looking to go for my HGV license so I can transport cars between the garages"
Smoke / Drink	"Don't smoke - does vaping count though? As for drinks, I have a few at the football and several with my mates after our football sesh"
VDU Use	"Use my phone a bit. Occasionally check the work one to sign off on jobs and print receipts, but I'd rather be tinkering, if I am honest!"
Contact Lenses	"Nah mate, not for me. I can't stand the thought of anything else in my eye"

Reflections on Case #017

Tentative Diagnosis: Right Eye: Metallic Foreign Body

Jack is fairly to the point and doesn't say too much. This could be just Jack's nature but also it could be because he is not feeling comfortable with the eye problem he has presented with. As this is his first memory of being in an optical setting, he may be confused with what happens during an appointment.

There are several points of interest in the case history that should be noted and understood. They may also contribute to Jack's management plan. Some areas of interest may be duplicate of previous cases. As such, I will highlight case-specific observations that may not have been covered on previous cases.

Suspect Foreign Body

Based on both the patient's history and symptoms, along with direct observation, it is highly likely that Jack has a foreign body in his eye. The sudden onset of symptoms while working on a car, immediately after feeling something enter the eye, strongly suggests this tentative diagnosis. Considering that he was working beneath a car, the probable foreign material is metallic.

Understanding the conditions of onset can provide clues about the type of foreign material:

- If the incident occurred in a garden, organic material may be involved, carrying a risk of fungal or other infections.

- In a dusty environment, the material could correspond to the composition of the dust.

- For someone grinding metal, the likely foreign body would indeed be metallic.

Different types of foreign bodies necessitate distinct management approaches. Therefore, asking questions related to the onset becomes particularly useful in reaching a working diagnosis.

Additionally, the speed of impact matters significantly. In Jack's case, it appears to be a low-impact foreign body, likely situated anteriorly. However, high-impact foreign bodies can potentially penetrate the globe, requiring further investigation and a referral.

While it may seem straightforward to acknowledge that the patient has something in their eye, delving into additional follow-up questions can significantly impact your management approach. Gather as much information as possible about the incident to guide your next steps effectively.

Management would also include a discussion on eye protection.

Case #018: James

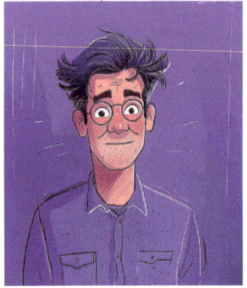

Composition – For the person acting as this patient:

James is a practical and focused 39-year-old workshop engineer. He initially sustained an eye injury 3 months ago, which seemed to heal. However, he has been experiencing recurrent episodes of eye pain and blurred vision, especially upon waking up in the morning.

The green text provides an example of the type of response you should provide to this question
Please note that this script spans two pages due to the "LOFTSEA" section.

Reason for Visit	"I keep getting recurring pain in my left eye, followed by blurring and light sensitivity. It's been on and off since I saw you a few months ago after that other incident"
Last Eye Examination	"I was seen here a few months back, was it 3 months or so? I think it was you that I saw"
Subjective Visual Assessment	"Vision has always been ok in glasses. When these episodes of pain occur, the left eye can be a bit blurry and watery"
Key Symptoms	"I wake up in the night to a sharp pain in the left eye, it stings like anything when it happens, then is watery and light sensitive. The next day it is blurry. It then heals but repeats again a few days later. It can feel a bit gritty, but no other noticeable symptoms I can tell you about"
LOFTSEA	
Location	"As I was saying, it was the left eye"
Onset	"Episodes on and off for the last month or so - think it could be related to that injury I had"
Frequency	"This morning was the 5th time it has happened, so definitely thought it would be worth getting checked out!"
Type	"Sharp, stabbing pain, approximately 7 out of 10 on the pain scale. Moderately watery as well"
Self Treatment	"I was using those dry eye drops you gave me, which don't do much during the day. The ointment for use at night was ok, but it makes my vision blurry, so no longer bother. Keeping my eyes shut eases the pain"
Effect on Life	"It's difficult to work when it happens as I need keen eyesight for my measurements. I'm exhausted if an episode starts at night!"
Associated	"Wateriness. No other discharge. It can also look very red when it happens and my wife wonders what is wrong with it!"

Ocular History	"That injury to the left eye, remember that belt buckle coming off of a conveyor belt and whacking me in the left eye? Thank you for getting me checked out at A&E - all ok with the retina and they said I had a lucky escape really as the injury could have been so much worse!" (No other known eye diseases, wears glasses for distance)
Family Ocular History	"Mum has iritis now and again, I have to take her to the hospital when it flares up. Dad died before I was born. No idea about the rest of the family" (No know other known eye diseases)
General Health	"I am a little overweight, but only just. Go to the gym regularly though." (No health complaints, no diabetes, no hypertension etc)
Medication	"Occasional hayfever tablet in the summer, when needed"
Allergies	"I occasionally get hayfever"
Family General Health	"Dad died young, as I was saying. Had a heart problem. I think he also had type 1 diabetes, but not sure. Everyone else is ok though!"
Hobbies/Interests	"Mountain biking, DIY projects - I have a fair few on the go right now, and I'm learning to play the guitar"
Driving Status	"I commute to work regularly by car. Always fancied learning to drive a bus, but went down the engineering route instead!"
Smoke / Drink	"No, I don't smoke. I like to have a beer or two in the evenings"
VDU Use	"I use it for moderate amounts of time. Couple of hours at work when designing something for the CAD modules and designing prints. Then just used for emails. These glasses do me fine and I am not having any issues"
Contact Lenses	"Not for me. Especially now I've got this eye problem. Never worn them and not looking to wear them either"

Reflections on Case #018

Tentative Diagnosis: Left Eye: Recurrent Epithelial Erosions Syndrome

James is a well spoken and articulate engineer that provides a great deal of information about his health, his symptoms and his history. Unlike many other presentations in this book, James has previously been seen by us for an assessment of the initial injury and as such this helps with further diagnosis of his presenting symptoms.

There are several points of interest in the case history that should be noted and understood. They may also contribute to James' management plan. Some areas of interest may be duplicate of previous cases. As such, I will highlight case-specific observations that may not have been covered on previous cases.

Recurrent Erosions

James is likely experiencing a recurrent epithelial erosion in his left eye. He recently sustained a traumatic injury in the left eye, causing corneal damage which is likely to have affected the basement membrane of his cornea meaning the epithelium is only loosely attached to the cornea. As the eyes dry slightly overnight, the epithelium adheres itself to the underside of the eyelid and is then sheared off when the eyelid opens, causing a large epithelial lesion that leads to acute, moderate to severe pain, watering and light sensitivity.

Given his recent traumatic history and the recurrent episodes having an onset upon waking, this is the likely tentative diagnosis.

Differential Diagnosis

James mentions that his mother experiences iritis, a form of uveitis. Interestingly, iritis shares some similarities with the tentative diagnosis of recurrent epithelial erosion. Both conditions present as painful, red eyes that are sensitive to light.

Now, let's address the question: Could this be iritis rather than recurrent epithelial erosion? The answer is: it's a possibility! While I emphasize the importance of the case history—often providing valuable clues even before the eye examination—it's essential to recognize that many eye conditions can resemble each other.

Why the Recurrent Epithelial Erosion Diagnosis?

- The case history highlights a previous eye injury, which could also trigger iritis.

- However, the specific pattern—short, sharp pain upon waking, followed by tearing and light sensitivity—aligns more closely with epithelial erosions.

In all cases, your assessment will be to document presence or absence of key signs in all likely cases to add evidence to or to rule out any given eye condition.

Treatment Compliance

In James' case, it appears that the previous appointment or eye casualty considered recurrent epithelial erosion as a possibility based on his current treatment regime. However, James is not following this regime because he doesn't believe it is effective, and the ointment's side effects discourage him from continued use.

Whenever a treatment plan is in effect—whether for recurrent epithelial erosion or any other condition—it is crucial to confirm patient compliance. Understanding whether the management is working or if the lack of response is due to non-compliance is essential.

Factors to Consider:

Patient Compliance: Investigate why James is non-compliant. Does he forget to follow the plan? Is he skeptical about its effectiveness (bearing in mind that some treatments may not yield immediate results)? Or are side effects hindering adherence?

Side Effects: In James' case, the ointment caused blurry vision. Advising him to apply it before sleep could mitigate this issue, as his eyes would be closed during that time and as such, blurriness would not be an issue.

Alternative Options: If non-compliance persists, explore alternative management strategies. Adjustments may be necessary to ensure effective treatment. Remember to always operate within your scope of practice and seek further advice if the management is beyond your remit.

Investigating the reasons behind non-compliance allows us to tailor management appropriately and find viable solutions.

Eye Protection

It has been mentioned in previous case studies, but does warrant being mentioned again here. If James has sustained an eye injury at work and he is still working in a similar environment following his injury, then make sure you have the discussion about safety glasses.

If he has them, remind him to wear them. If he doesn't have any, discuss with him the importance of having some to prevent a repeat of his experience and/or experiencing other forms of ocular injury in the future.

It is likely this was done on his initial presentation, but given he was rushed to A&E, this advice was probably low on his immediate priority list and may have been forgotten about. Take the time to remind him today!

Case #019: Sarah

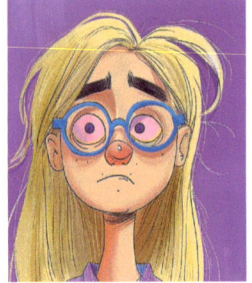

Composition – For the person acting as this patient:

Sarah is a 45-year-old cleaner who is experiencing symptoms consistent with an eye infection. She has a history of health anxiety, which exacerbates her concern about her symptoms and their implications. She is seeking reassurance and effective treatment. Be intense in your answering.

The green text provides an example of the type of response you should provide to this question
Please note that this script spans two pages due to the "LOFTSEA" section.

Reason for Visit	"Both my eyes are really red and sore. I think both my retinas are detaching and I'm really scared. I think the retinas are coming out through my eyes as there's this yellow gunky stuff on my eyelids!"
Last Eye Examination	"4 months ago. I really ought to be seen monthly as worried my eyes will go the same way as my mum's did, but I've been told I need an eye exam every two years""
Subjective Visual Assessment	"Really blurry when the yellow stuff goes over my eyes. I can just about manage for distance without glasses but reading is a must. Although I don't like wearing glasses as they weaken the eyes!"
Key Symptoms	"Redness, itchiness, gritty feeling in the eyes, and yellowish discharge that crusts the eyelashes, especially when I woke up" (No headaches, diplopia or flashes or floaters - but if asked, press to ask what those symptoms mean and push for why they are being asked)
LOFTSEA	
Location	"As you can see, it's both my eyes"
Onset	"Started this morning. Why I had to wait until this afternoon to be seen, I don't know. The delay has likely caused me to lose my sight permanently!"
Frequency	"Not gotten any better since I woke up with it. Constantly there affecting my eyes!"
Type	"It's really uncomfortable and gritty. This yellow discharge shows no sign of stopping. It's my retinas. I just know it!"
Self Treatment	"I tried bathing it with warm water and wiping away the discharge. It helps but I'm worried I'm going to do harm without advice!"
Effect on Life	"It's playing on my health anxiety. I mean, this is it, isn't it? 45 years young and I'm going to lose my sight!!"
Associated	"I'm terrified my retinas are going to spread to my family and cause it to happen to them. It is really worrying me!"

Ocular History	"I never have had this before. But I am aware my eyesight is gradually getting worse each year and of late I cannot see very well up close. Frustratingly, I feel these glasses you sold me are making things worse." (No other known eye diseases, wears glasses for distance and reading)
Family Ocular History	"Mum has glaucoma and she also had a retinal detachment. I think I recall her having symproms like this. I can't remember!" (No know other known eye diseases)
General Health	"I get significant palpitations. I swear it is a heart problem, but I keep getting fobbed off and told that it is anxiety. That said, I am aware that I have health anxiety. No diabetes or anything, but I swear it is coming! That and other diseases that come with age!" (No other health complaints, no diabetes, no hypertension, not pregnant or breastfeeding)
Medication	"Sertraline and propranolol. Occasional diazepam when anxiety becomes crippling."
Allergies	"Dustmites, cats, dogs, horses, guinea pigs and latex"
Family General Health	"Mum has diabetes. I knew it. Its the family history coming in. You're going to find diabetes, aren't you?"
Hobbies/Interests	"Reading, gardening, and yoga."
Driving Status	"I drive, but don't think I am in any fit state to with my eyes like this!"
Smoke / Drink	"No to both"
VDU Use	"I heard that computer screens ruin your eyes so try and use one as little as possible. I take bookings via email, so that is all I use it for. Probably about 30 mins a day at most!"
Contact Lenses	"Not worn them. Glasses are bad enough, don't want anything else to cause me eye problems!"

Reflections on Case #019

Tentative Diagnosis: Bilateral Bacterial Conjunctivitis

Sarah is a anxious patient that suffers with health anxiety. Her signs and symptoms indicate a bilateral conjunctivitis and with the type of discharge produced, it is likely to be bacterial in origin. Managing her health anxiety will be more of a challenge than the presenting ocular condition.

There are several points of interest in the case history that should be noted and understood. They may also contribute to Sarah's management plan. Some areas of interest may be duplicate of previous cases. As such, I will highlight case-specific observations that may not have been covered on previous cases.

Health Anxiety

Health anxiety is a psychological condition where an individual experiences persistent worries and fears about having (or developing) undiagnosed medical conditions. These anxieties can become so intense that they can interfere with a person's quality of life.

They may exhibit signs of constant worry, be seeking reassurance that all is ok, be prone to doing excessive research of conditions on the internet or even demonstrate physical symptoms of anxiety that may cause them to think they have an illness (such as headaches, palpitations and tremors).

In this case, you will need to manage the patient's health anxiety alongside the presenting complaint. Here are some tips on managing a patient with an eye condition when they demonstrate (or provide diagnosis of) health anxiety:

- **Validate their feelings.** Let them know it is common to feel worried about health issues. This validation helps create a safe place for discussion, whilst allowing you to build trust with the patient.

- **Empathise and encourage.** Demonstrate empathy and encourage your patient to be open with their fears. Let them feel seen, heard and understood. Try hard to dispel the fears (i.e. In Sarah's case, whilst we know the yellow discharge is not her retinas detaching through her tears, don't scoff at her and be constructive in your explanation of what it is).

- **Be clear and avoid jargon.** Use simple language and be clear in any explanations provided. Try not to provide more information than is necessary for the case as this may fuel further health anxieties (e.g. in this case stick to the management plan for bacterial conjunctivitis and don't start with treatments about retinal tears and detachments if you've already ruled out there isn't one).

- **Recap and questions.** Remember to recap essential information to reinforce understanding and allow time to answer any further queries or uncertainties that your patient has.

Red Eye

Red eyes can have a range of different causes (scelritis, iritis, conjunctivitis, episcleritis, contact lens induced red eye, keratitis, dry eye, subconjunctival haemorrhage, blepharitis, photokeratitis, chemical injury and foreign bodies to name just a few!)

For this case scenario, the basics were covered to follow on with the key format of the case scenario. Whilst some of the additional questions arise through general LOFTSEA questioning, further red eye questions should be asked for any patient presenting with red eyes. These questions include:

- **Discharge.** Knowing if the eye has discharge can help remove non-discharge producing differential diagnoses. Asking the patient to describe the discharge can help identify the cause (mucopurulent can indicate bacterial, watery could be viral etc.)

- **Contact lens use.** Knowing if a patient wears contact lenses can help identify if it is a contact lens related problem. Investigating their compliance and hygiene can further narrow down on suspected tentative diagnoses.

- **Foreign body.** Asking if the patient has felt anything go into their eye could help lead to a work up where a foreign body could be present. Knowing the speed it entered the eye can help provide further information on whether or not to suspect a penetrating eye injury.

- **Trauma.** Blunt trauma can lead to subconjunctival haemorrhages or lacerations lead to anterior eye inflammation which will produce redness of the eye(s). Knowing if trauma is present, as well as the type, will help you perform further appropriate investigations of the retina and orbit.

- **Systemic health conditions**. Some systemic health conditions can be a risk factor for a specific range of red eyes (e.g. arthritis and it's associated conditions can be a risk factor of other inflammatory eye diseases such as uveitis and episcleritis). Asking further questions regarding health when a tentative diagnosis has formed can further add weight to your diagnosis.

- **Recent health issues**. Recent respiratory infections such as colds or covid can lead to viral conjunctivitis, or even bacterial conjunctivitis as the illness lowers the patient's immune system.

- **Recent cold sores.** Herpes simplex keratitis can occur in patients that have cold sores - although can also occur in patients without them.

- **Other systemic signs.** The patient may report fever, rashes or other illnesses that have no official diagnoses. For instance, a patient with a rash on their face may have signs of shingles (herpes zoster that may be affecting the eye.

Whilst this list is long, it is not exhaustive. Ask as many appropriate questions as you need to help build a case to back your working diagnoses.

Case #020: Jordan

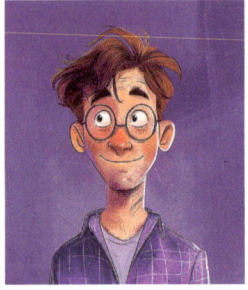

Composition – For the person acting as this patient:

Jordan is a 32-year-old freelance graphic designer who has had a recent diagnosis of multiple sclerosis. He is relatively friendly and talkative, despite being in some discomfort with his symptoms.

The green text provides an example of the type of response you should provide to this question

Please note that this script spans two pages due to the "LOFTSEA" section.

Reason for Visit	"My left eye is quite uncomfortable when I look around. I really don't know why. The vision also isn't too good - it's slightly patchy and I also get like a second image when I look around"
Last Eye Examination	"Probably about 6 months ago at the place down the street from here"
Subjective Visual Assessment	"When I look up, I see sort of two of everything, you know, side by side? My vision was otherwise ok about a week ago, but the vision is the left eye feels a bit patchy at all distances"
Key Symptoms	"As I was saying, the vision is a bit patchy in the left, the eye hurts when I look around and I get double vision when I look up" (No headaches, flashes or floaters)
LOFTSEA	
Location	"It's my left eye. The double vision goes if I close it"
Onset	"Vision in the left eye started going a bit patchy a few days ago, the doubling happened this morning, along with the eye ache - so I was advised by my doctor to have an eye test"
Frequency	"I mean, it's been there since it started, but the intensity fluctuates quite a bit!"
Type	"Well, moderate discomfort on eye movement, unusual patchy vision in the left eye and horizontal double vision when I look up"
Self Treatment	"These symptoms seem complex. I don't really know where to start on easing them! I have found keeping my eyes still helps with the discomfort though"
Effect on Life	"I'm not able to work so well. It's quite uncomfortable and when I am working I don't know what image to look at!"
Associated	"I feel fairly fatigued at the moment, but I am not sure if that is my MS playing up or the stress of these symptoms"

Ocular History	"I wear my glasses all the time mostly, as I am slightly short-sighted. I've not been told that I have any eye conditions at the moment but was advised I may have eye problems from time to time after my diagnosis of multiple sclerosis" (No other eye diseases known, no trips to the hospital eye service)
Family Ocular History	"Mum has glaucoma and I think my nan had that thing where they had to inject stuff in her eyeballs for, what's it called? Oh yeah, molecular degenerations"
General Health	"I was diagnosed with multiple sclerosis about 6 months ago, so that has had a significant effect on my life. I am currently taking medication that has it under control though, although I do feel fatigued, so may have to speak the doctor again. I also have anxiety, of which is heightened when I have a flare up of MS symptoms, which I do actually feel is happening now!" (No other health complaints, no diabetes, no hypertension etc)
Medication	"Cladribine, for the MS and sertraline for anxiety"
Allergies	"I'm a coeliac, but no other known allergies"
Family General Health	"My grandfather had a stroke when he was 75, dad has diabetes and mum recently has been told she has high blood pressure"
Hobbies/Interests	"Painting, hiking and photography, although it's been a tough few months so I haven't managed to do it as much as I'd like"
Driving Status	"I drive a car occasionally. I think I'm legal to drive without glasses but wouldn't ever risk it!"
Smoke / Drink	"No to both"
VDU Use	"I have to use it quite a bit for work and also when I edit my photos. I would say I probably need to use it over 8 hours a day, 10+ if you count the amount of time on my phone!"
Contact Lenses	"Oh yeah, I wear them!"
Further CL Details	ONLY GIVE THE BELOW INFORMATION WHEN ASKED
Lens Type	"The Advocate Breathe 1-Day"
Age of Current Lenses	"I'm not wearing any"
Average Wear Time	"2-3 hours socially, no more than twice a month"
Solutions Used	"No solutions - I bin them when I take them out"
Swimming in Lenses?	"No"
Showering in Lenses?	"No"
Sleeping in Lenses?	"No"
Last time you wore lenses?	"About 3 weeks ago"
Any problems?	"Nope, they're comfortable and I see well out of them"

Reflections on Case #020

Tentative Diagnosis: Left Eye Optic Neuritis

Jordan is a pleasant patient that, whilst in some discomfort with his symptoms, is happy to answer and interact with you to find a source of his complaints

There are several points of interest in the case history that should be noted and understood. They may also contribute to Jordan's management plan. Some areas of interest may be duplicate of previous cases. As such, I will highlight case-specific observations that may not have been covered on previous cases.

Optic Neuritis

The most likely diagnosis here is optic neuritis and, whilst a full work up would be required prior to managing (in this case an urgent referral to ophthalmology), there may be many tests that you would like to run to aid your colleagues in the ophthalmology department.

The case history indicates Jordan has multiple sclerosis (MS) which is a neurological condition that can affect the nerves of the body, including the ones responsible for the function of the eye. One of the ways that multiple sclerosis can first be suspected is through a case of optic neuritis, which is inflammation of the optic nerve.

Common symptoms of optic neuritis are:
- Vision loss
- Loss of colour vision
- Discomfort and diplopia on eye movements
- Reduction in contrast sensitivity

Jordan also reports some of the above symptoms as his reason for visit.

If you suspect a case of optic neuritis (or other neurological findings), it is essential to ensure that you perform colour vision testing to assess for red desaturation, visual fields testing for field defects and pupil assessment to assess for relative afferent pupillary defects.

Being able to select the most appropriate tests following a case history is vital in your planning of the appointment and the tests chosen should aim to maximise the information gained in the time you have to see the patient.

General Health

This case also gives extra strength to the importance of taking account of the patient's general health, as the history of multiple sclerosis significantly weights the tentative diagnosis towards optic neuritis. Furthermore, the patient stating that they are having a flare up of symptoms would strengthen this tentative diagnosis further.

Contact Lenses

Jordan is also a contact lens wearer, a detail that might have been overlooked without your thorough questioning. While not necessarily significant in this specific case, having this additional knowledge can help explain any additional findings and rule out other potential diagnoses.

In Jordan's situation, he is a compliant and low-risk lens wearer, making it highly unlikely that contact lenses are the cause of his symptoms. However, when referring him, it's essential to mention his contact lens use. Additionally, inform him about potential treatments for optic neuritis, such as topical steroids. It's crucial to emphasise that wearing lenses during treatment would be contraindicated, and he should avoid them until the treatment is completed

Driving

Jordan has mentioned that he drives with corrective lenses. Additionally, he believes he meets the legal requirements to drive without glasses, although he chooses not to do so. It's common for patients to assert that their vision is "just fine" for driving, whether they wear corrective lenses or not. As an optometrist, it's essential to assess whether their vision truly meets the legal standard based on their habitual way of driving.

In Jordan's case, I would also perform an acuity measurement without his glasses. Based on the results, I can provide a definitive answer:

- If his vision falls below the legal standard, I would recommend that he wears glasses while driving.

- If his vision meets the legal requirements, I can inform him that he is technically okay to drive without glasses but would be able to see clearer/further away/better with them.

Clear communication of these findings ensures that patients like Jordan understand their options and can make informed decisions regarding their driving habits.

Closing Notes on Case Study Selection 3

This section delved into a variety of different presentations of eye pain and discomfort; from the emergency scenarios through to those with chronic pain that need further management from you. These cases are usually seen via locally accredited schemes (such as the Minor Eye Care Scheme (MECS) or Coronavirus Urgent Eye Service (CUES)) so you may not see many of these unless you are accredited to perform these services or work in an area without them.

Whilst these cases will be managed differently to a routine appointment, these case histories are vital to help establish a differential diagnosis of their presenting complaints. Performing practice sessions with these case notes will allow you to understand where you need to focus your questions to keep the appointment relevant for that patient.

Reason for Visit There were a range of different presenting concerns that centred around a painful or uncomfortable eye. Taking the time to establish the concerns and the relevant information to form a thorough history will help you tentatively diagnose the issue and allow you to ask the appropriate follow up questions (such as contact-lens specific questions that will help point to the cause of their symptoms. It will also aid your ability to select the most appropriate tests to investigate their symptoms further.

Health and Family Clues As mentioned before, the health of a patient and their family history can help guide you to the tentative diagnosis. A diagnosis of multiple sclerosis and the relevant symptoms being described indicate optic neuritis; or Sarah's revelation that she has had a recent cold and suffers from health anxiety will really help guide you to that tentative diagnosis.

Glasses Talk While refractive issues were less prominent in these cases, the need for corrective eyewear as part of the management plan was evident in cases such as #016, where Morgan's contact lens misuse could be addressed. A discussion on a careful dispense with high index lenses and a smaller frame may tackle her concerns on spectacle wear and encourage safe contact lens use.

Contact Lens Chat

The cases involving contact lenses underscored the importance of appropriate contact lens education. We should always be encouraging contact lens wearers to use their lenses appropriately and address areas of risk. Whilst it may be too late to tackle the presenting problem, reminding them the likely cause is the consequences of lens abuse will stay strong in their minds. Furthermore, whenever a patient presents with a painful and/or red eye, it is important to know their history with contact lenses – asking further questions on their use will often pinpoint the cause of their complaints.

Patient Emotions

The emotional states of patients, such as the health anxiety experienced by Sarah and the onset of conjunctivitis, or the exhausted presentation of Morgan with her acanthamoeba keratitis, show that we need to be adaptive to our patients. You may need to modify your approach to gather all the information you need, but always remain objective, empathetic and avoid being judgemental – remember, you are there to help!

In summary, these cases illustrate the nature of eye care, where understanding the patient's lifestyle, emotional state, and medical history is as crucial as the clinical examination itself. Practitioners must adapt their approach to each unique scenario, ensuring that patient concerns are met with both technical expertise and compassionate care.

Closing Notes

Optometric case histories are the cornerstone for every eye examination and episode of patient care. They provide a detailed account of a patient's visual and medical history. offering insights that are crucial for accurate diagnosis and effective treatment plans. This study guide equipped optometry students with the knowledge and skills necessary to conduct thorough case histories, ensuring they are well-prepared for clinical practice, whilst providing food for thought for seasoned professionals looking to keep their skills sharp.

Learning the right questions to ask is an art that all optometry students must master. This guide outlined the types of questions that elicit the most informative responses, from general health inquiries to specific ocular symptoms. It emphasises the importance of open-ended questions and active listening to understand the patient's concerns fully.

The book contained 20 diverse scripts that simulate real-life scenarios optometrists may encounter. These scripts range from routine check-ups to complex cases involving systemic diseases with ocular manifestations. Each script was followed by an analysis section, guiding you through the reasoning behind each question and the significance of the responses received. Whilst the full extent of each encounter was not able to be fully investigated, each key point provided a pearl of clinical wisdom from which to build clinical understanding and encourage reflective practice.

Analysing patient responses is as important as asking the right questions. This guide provided strategies for interpreting answers and identifying red flags that may indicate underlying conditions. It also discusses how to piece together information to form a comprehensive picture of the patient's ocular and systemic health.

The study guide reinforces the idea that proficiency in taking optometric case histories is achieved through practice and reflection. It encourages students to use the scripts provided to hone their skills and to continually seek out new learning opportunities.

I hope this study guide has been of use to you and if so, please consider leaving us a review and recommendation. All feedback is welcome and will be used to help create further study guides in the future.

Many thanks again for purchasing and all the best in your endeavours into the world of optometry!

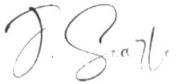

Further Reading

The following further reading suggestions are resources that I have found useful over the years and through the production of this Study Guide. You may wish to visit these resources to further understand the topic of optometric case history taking.

Geeky Medics: Ophthalmic History Taking - OSCE Guide

This guide, aimed at medical and ophthalmology students gives a complete rundown of an ophthalmic case history taking within the OSCE format. It is useful for students and pre-registration optometrists to understand what would be expected from them during an OSCE or SOPE station.

https://geekymedics.com/ophthalmic-history-taking-osce-guide/

Review of Optometry: Developing a Constructive Approach to Case History

This article, aimed at US-based optometrists covers how to take a detailed and thorough case history within the optometric setting. Whilst primarily geared for a US-based system, many tips can be taken for effective UK-based assessments too. Additionally, it is useful to see how different systems across the world work and the differences within the roles between UK and US optometrists.

https://www.reviewofoptometry.com/article/developing-a-constructive-approach-to-case-history

College of Optometrists: What to Record

This professional guidance is useful to read through as it will give you the information on what you MUST record during a case history and what you SHOULD record. Note the differences in terminology and make sure the MUST records are recorded on each examination at the very least/

https://www.college-optometrists.org/clinical-guidance/guidance/knowledge,-skills-and-performance/patient-records#Whattorecord

About the Author

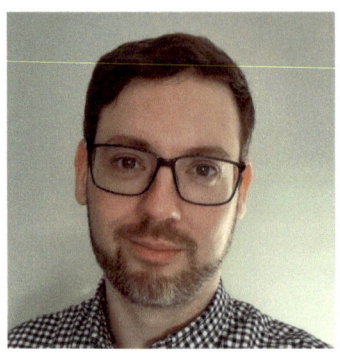

Jason Searle

Jason Searle is an accomplished optometrist with extensive experience in the field. Graduating in 2013, and subsequently qualifying in 2014, he quickly established himself as a trusted professional within optometry clinics. Over the years, he has held various roles within optics, ophthalmology and academia, gaining valuable insights into patient care.

Since 2014, Jason has been working as a locum optometrist, contributing his expertise to more than 50 practices. His adaptability and commitment to excellence have made him a sought-after optometrist within the South West of England and the South East of Wales.

Beyond clinical practice, Jason is the founder of The Eye Care Advocate, a platform dedicated to promoting eye health awareness and education. His passion for advocacy extends to teaching and supervising optometry students at the undergraduate level.

With a wealth of knowledge and a genuine desire to improve eye health, Jason brings a unique perspective to the field. His dedication to patient well-being and professional growth makes him an asset to the optometric community.

www.theeyecareadvocate.co.uk

Acknowledgements

I just wanted to add a few words of acknowledgement to those that helped inspire and encourage me to create this study guide.

To my wife, Hannah, thank you for convincing me to stick with this project through to completion and for your patience whilst I spent countless hours typing, formatting and editing the content. I'll definitely be thankful for the time you spent proofreading the final draft to have it ready for publication.

To my son, Arthur. I appreciate you coming in to my office to see how much I have progressed with the study guide - and for providing me with tasks that gave me valid breaks from typing and working!

Additionally, a special thank you to the staff and students of the University of West of England's optometry department:

To the staff, thank you for taking me on board and for the encouragement to work within a teaching role. Out of all the roles I have had, my time supervising undergraduates has been my favourite.

To the students, thank you for being so inspirational. You may have learned things from me, but I have certainly learned things from you too! I look forward to working alongside you all when you qualify and just hope you won't be put off hiring me as one of your locum optometrists,

www.ingramcontent.com/pod-product-compliance
Lightning Source LLC
Chambersburg PA
CBHW040220220526
45473CB00001B/59

of it, and can be significantly dependent on both personal or professional relationships, and confidence."[4] *The Economic Times* defines negotiation as essentially "an exchange of dialogues involving two or maybe more conflicting parties who are striving to reach a consensus on their dilemma."[5] The *Financial Times* published an article emphasizing that negotiation "is more than a technical skill…It is a core component of leadership."[6]

Another aspect to keep in mind is that negotiations exist on multiple levels: interpersonal, team, organizational, and even in virtual space. Additionally, negotiation is influenced by various antecedents, including personal, emotional, contextual, and organizational factors.

While numerous definitions of negotiation exist, here's the one that will be used throughout the book, informed by extensive negotiation experience and a comprehensive review of negotiation literature: *Negotiation is a process of communication where two or more parties analyze alternatives with the aim of achieving a shared decision.* In other words, negotiation doesn't necessarily require any conflict or contradiction between parties. So there are three conditions to make a negotiation happen: two or more parties, a consensus to be achieved, a set of alternatives to be discussed. If one or more of these three conditions is missing, there can't be a negotiation.

Overall, we can draw several conclusions from our discussion so far. First, negotiation encompasses a number of elements: a shared decision, different interests, common ground, joint agreement, an acceptable solution, win-win situations, an outcome that suits all parties. In other words, in a successful negotiation, there are no winners and losers, but there is agreement and a certain level of satisfaction for all parties (although this may vary). What's brought to the table are often different interests and positions, sometimes conflicting with each other, but the result should be a shared solution that suits all parties. Second, in successful negotiations, when the parties achieve an outcome that addresses their interests, they experience satisfaction. We'll look at this behavioral-emotional dimension of negotiation in more detail in Chapter 4. Third, negotiation is defined as a learning process, a technical method, and a component of leadership. This means negotiation is a skill that can be learned, a process that can be comprehended, with techniques for success that can be mastered.

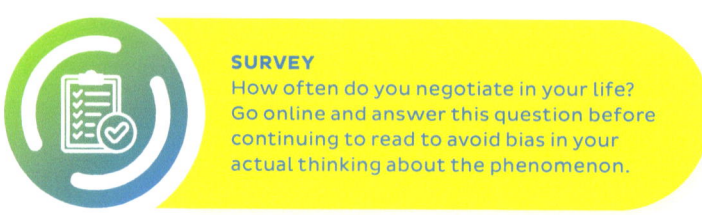

SURVEY
How often do you negotiate in your life? Go online and answer this question before continuing to read to avoid bias in your actual thinking about the phenomenon.

1.2 HOW OFTEN DO WE ACTUALLY NEGOTIATE?

> Good heavens! For more than forty years I have been speaking prose without knowing it.
>
> – Molière, *The Bourgeois Gentleman*, 1670

Having defined negotiation, the next question that arises is: How often do we negotiate? According to *Forbes*, we negotiate every day, in situations where our interests with another person or company diverge (or partially diverge) and we are looking for an agreement, with the family, with the insurance company, with the team at work when they are not too supportive of your idea.[7]

Negotiations influence both our personal and professional lives in many ways. Let's consider the following examples in the personal sphere. Your teenage daughter wants to travel abroad with her friends. You find yourself concerned about her safety but reluctant to refuse her permission outright. So the two of you would negotiate to find a solution that allows her to enjoy the trip while ensuring her safety and alleviating your worries. Another example: You might take your clothes to the drycleaner and ask them to expedite the service, explaining that you need your suit for an important conference. Your request would prompt them to complete the job in short order.

So, whether it's a family deciding on a show to watch in the evening or choosing a country for their next vacation, or a shopper haggling over the price of vegetables at the market, or a homebuyer securing a mortgage with a bank, to achieve the best possible deal, negotiation is a common part of everyday life that happens frequently in a variety of situations.

Indeed, in business life negotiation is also a regular occurrence. When offered a new position, you may negotiate your KPIs, the resources you need to achieve your objectives, and your salary. In day-to-day work, negotiations are common when deciding how tasks will be allocated within a team or whether deadlines can be adjusted.

All in all, negotiation is an integral phenomenon of our daily personal and professional lives.

1.3 COMMON MISPERCEPTIONS AROUND NEGOTIATION

Often, we think we're not involved in a negotiation because of some misperceptions, that is, misunderstandings or fundamental errors in judgment. Drawing on the literature on the subject, here are some very common misperceptions that inform our idea of negotiation.

- *There's a winner and a loser – and nobody wants to lose.* In fact, negotiation is often perceived in win-lose terms, with the assumption that if one side is winning, the other side is losing. However, this is far removed from the true nature of negotiation, where the aim should be to foster long-term relationships and potential cooperation. If there is a loser, that person will be less inclined to build a long-term relationship. In addition, the essence of negotiation is to find an answer that satisfies all parties, making creative solutions a crucial component.
- *Compromise is a false promise.* Here the erroneous notion is that to come to an agreement, someone has to sacrifice something important. This leads to compromise, which often leaves all parties in the negotiation somewhat dissatisfied. Such an approach can be risky, as unresolved dissatisfaction may lead to conflict, potentially resulting in further negotiations or, at worst, a solution that is highly unfavorable to one or more parties.
- *Negotiation always involves manipulation.* Negotiation should exclude manipulation and instead focus on finding mutually satisfactory solutions through creativity, cooperation, and collaborative problem-solving. Feeling manipulated leaves people with a sense of uneasiness, mistrust; it creates a negative atmosphere, and leads to the failure of the negotiation or to the dissolution of the partnership, temporarily or even permanently.
- *Negotiation is for the weak.* When discussing negotiation, we often refer

to strong and weak positions. A strong position is characterized by compelling arguments, sizeable resources, and the power to sway decisions. Conversely, a weak position is defined by the lack of persuasive arguments, a limited range of options, and few or no resources. In fact, the thinking is that if you're in a strong position, there's no need to negotiate. This misconception is a drastic mistake, illustrated by many examples from history, politics, and business. Overall, a strong position is not the same as having a strong negotiating party, and even here it's beneficial to negotiate because it helps to form a coalition of like-minded people, create an atmosphere of trust, and gain broad support.
- *Negotiating to achieve short-term contractual goals comes at the cost of long-term relationships.* This represents a misperception because preserving the long-term relationship is an essential task. It helps pave the way for new initiatives, strengthen existing projects, build the foundation for establishing long-term cooperation and exploring new opportunities.
- *Overestimating the strength of the other party* is a frequent occurrence in business contexts. This misjudgment can be driven by various factors, such as that company's size, its reputation for tough negotiations, or the status of its brand. But these perceptions are often more subjective and emotionally driven than grounded in reality. The size of a company does not necessarily dictate the outcome of negotiations on a particular issue. In such situations, it's crucial to accurately assess information about the other party, recognize your own strengths, and not be intimidated by the other side's brand or reputation.
- *Overconfidence* is the exact opposite of the previous point. In this scenario, one side overestimates its resources, negotiation skills, and the solidity of its arguments. This can create the illusion that there is no need to prepare for the negotiation. Also, overconfidence can encourage a party to be aggressive and greedy. This can lead to negative consequences, up to and including losing the negotiation.
- *The art of negotiation cannot be learned.* Many people believe that the ability to negotiate successfully is a gift that they can't learn. Instead, it's a skill that can be acquired and developed.

In general, understanding and recognizing the key misperceptions described above can significantly increase the chances of success in negotiations.

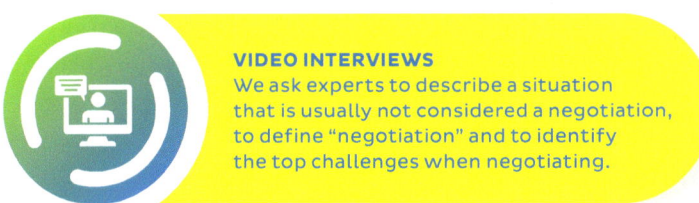

VIDEO INTERVIEWS
We ask experts to describe a situation that is usually not considered a negotiation, to define "negotiation" and to identify the top challenges when negotiating.

1.4 GAME THEORY

Game theory attracts the attention not only of business professionals, economists, and scientists but also creative people, as evidenced by films such as *A Beautiful Mind* and *Hidden Figures*, which explore its basic concepts. Game theory extends beyond traditional boundaries, finding applications in card games, chess, politics, economics, trade, corporate processes, and even personal relationships. In the context of negotiations, game theory serves as a valuable tool, as it involves the study of optimal strategies in competitive and collaborative scenarios.

A game is understood as an interaction among two or more parties, each with their own interests. In this sense, a game is a very common situation – any interaction with someone else, at work, in your family, in everyday life can be considered as a game. The peculiarity of the game is that the outcome is contingent not only on your actions and decisions, but also on the actions and decisions of the other participant(s). So the end result depends on how well you understand and predict the actions of the other player(s). Beyond understanding their strategy, you also have to develop an appropriate response to their actions.

Additionally, in game theory there are several initial conditions-assumptions. Each participant in the game has several choices in terms of actions, and all actions affect all players. What's more, all participants are rational and make decisions based on rational arguments and information. But here's the rub: In real life, people are not always rational. And this applies not only to family life, but also to business relations, politics, and so on. As a result, many strategies fail because another player can make decisions based on emotional or subjective states. (See Chapter 4 to explore the emotional aspect of negotiations.)

Returning to game theory, it's worthwhile to highlight several key concepts. Let's delve into some of them, starting with the Nash equilibrium. This is a scenario in which a player can't gain any advantage by changing their strategy unless the other player changes theirs too. So equilibrium is beneficial and stable, but a change of strategy can lead to losses.

There are also scenarios where both sides win or both lose. The prisoner's dilemma is a classic case in which each player must decide whether to work with or against the other, with the outcome hinging on both players' strategies. However, neither player knows the other's decision in advance. If both sides choose to cooperate, they achieve the best possible outcome. But if one betrays the other, both parties lose. In the context of negotiation, the prisoner's dilemma illustrates how people may refrain from cooperating, or even abandon negotiations altogether, despite the fact that working together would potentially yield the most favorable results for everyone involved.

In zero-sum games, if one player wins, the other loses. For example, when bidding on a contract that can only be awarded to one company, it's a case of winner-takes-all, while the other party receives nothing.

Some games have simultaneous moves when players make decisions and take actions at the same time, without knowing the strategy of the other player. In contrast, in sequential games, players take turns, like in chess. This gives them the opportunity to observe and react to the strategies of other players before making their own move. In this way, a competitor can adjust their initial strategy by drawing conclusions based on another player's previous moves. There are also repetitive games in which the decisions of players in a new game are influenced by their experience of interaction with their opponent in previous games.

Game theory highlights several vital issues, one of which is the importance of collaboration. In certain types of games, cooperation can significantly impact the outcome, often leading to beneficial results for all. Another key issue is the role of information. In games with sequential moves, information becomes crucial, as it allows players to interpret the actions of others and shape their strategies accordingly. Moreover, in repetitive or iterative games, trust becomes a vital factor, as players base their decisions on the outcomes and behaviors observed in previous rounds.

In addition to games with individual players, there are games played in groups. Here there is a different logic and, as seen in the literature, the decisions of a group are less rational than those of an individual. For example, a group may opt for a given course of action not because it seems to be the right way to go, but because the majority of the group will agree. A good illustration here is the classic case of the Keynesian beauty contest, in which the members of the jury don't choose the individual they personally find most beautiful. Instead, they try to guess which contestant would be considered the most beautiful by most of the other judges because they want to join the majority opinion. In negotiations we often encounter group decisions, e.g., a team discussing the criteria to make certain choices, managers preparing to deliver some news, a group of companies debating on how to move forward on a joint project.

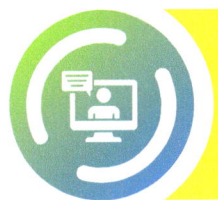

VIDEO INTERVIEWS
How do you negotiate effectively?
We encourage you to answer this question before watching the next series of video interviews and hearing the experts' perspectives.

1.5 KEY PRINCIPLES OF EFFECTIVE NEGOTIATORS

What clearly emerges from the previous sections is that learning to negotiate effectively requires considerable work and training. The starting point is to have a very good understanding of some basic principles of negotiation. Based on an extensive literature review, below are seven principles adopted by effective negotiators which we'll explore in-depth in the following chapters of the book.

Successful negotiation hinges on thorough *preparation* (see Chapter 2). By preparation we mean both planning for the negotiation process itself and gaining a deep understanding of the other people at the table. Being well-prepared means having a clear objective, identifying a strategy to achieve it, anticipating potential objections from others, and planning how to respond to these objections. Preparation also includes gathering information and analyzing data about all parties. However, when information is limited, alternative approaches, such as modeling and predicting, can be applied. Additionally, good preparation increases confidence, leads to advantageous outcomes, and fosters effective negotiation.

When negotiating, a fundamental principle is *creative problem solving* (see Chapter 2). The challenge that lies at the heart of negotiation is attempting to unite interests that are not so well aligned and may even be conflicting. Taking this into account, it is crucial to maintain long-term relationships, to build trust between the parties, and to create a foundation for further cooperation. In these circumstances, creativity is an invaluable skill for negotiators. A creative approach to decision-making provides opportunities to embrace shared values instead of fueling conflict. Overall, creativity takes the relationship to a new level while achieving the goal of the negotiation.

Being ready to *walk away* is the next principle of effective negotiators (see Chapter 3). This means that in some scenarios, it's better to stop negotiating than to agree to terms you are not satisfied with. Obviously, this doesn't mean you should be inflexible, but you need to keep your balance and decide ahead of time when you would do better to walk away.

Managing the *emotional side* of negotiation is a very essential principle (see Chapter 4). Clearly, emotions can both help and hinder the success of negotiations. In any case, it's vital to control this side of negotiation processes; neglecting emotions can be a serious mistake. Today more and more attention is being paid to emotional intelligence, with studies showing that it has become a priority in business.

Another major principle of negotiation is *clear and effective communication* (see Chapter 5). It's crucial to deliver your arguments clearly to ensure the other party understands you. However, this seemingly obvious principle is often overlooked. Frequently, the parties involved fail to clearly deliver pertinent information; arguments are not effectively communicated, and explanations may be either lacking or unclear. In addition, communication includes a non-verbal component. This means it's essential to make sure that your gestures and facial expressions are in line with the objectives of the negotiation and send the right signal to the other party.

Effective negotiators know how important it is to *uncover hidden areas* of negotiation (see Chapters 2 and 6). Research shows that many antecedences influence negotiation, including gender, age, emotional state, and previous experience, as well as cultural differences, habits, and traditions. International negotiation, for example, is a separate area that requires extensive training (Chapter 6).

Being prepared to negotiate in both physical and *digital settings* is also relevant in today's context (Chapter 7).

In the next chapter, we'll walk you through the negotiation process, including understanding, acting, and reviewing it.

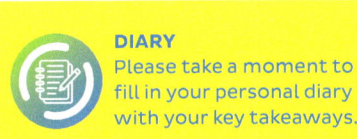

DIARY
Please take a moment to fill in your personal diary with your key takeaways.

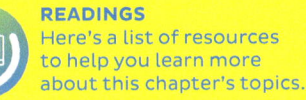

READINGS
Here's a list of resources to help you learn more about this chapter's topics.

SUMMARY

DEFINITION OF NEGOTIATION	• Academic perspective • Practice perspective • Author's perspective: Negotiation is a process of communication where two or more parties analyze alternatives with the aim of achieving a shared decision.
MISPERCEPTIONS OF NEGOTIATION	• A winner and a loser – and nobody wants to lose • False promise of compromise • Negotiation always involves manipulation. • Negotiation is for the weak. • Negotiate to achieve short-term contractual goals at the cost of long-term relationships • Overestimate the strength of the other party • Overconfidence • The art of negotiation cannot be learned.
GAME THEORY	• The Nash equilibrium • The prisoner's dilemma • Zero-sum games
KEY PRINCIPLES OF EFFECTIVE NEGOTIATION	• Preparation • Creative problem solving • Willingness to walk away • Control of the emotional side • Clear and effective communication • Uncover hidden areas • Being ready for the phygital setting

NOTES

[1] Henry A. Kissinger, "The Vietnam Negotiations," *Survival* 11, no. 2 (February 1969): 38–50, https://doi.org/10.1080/00396336908440951.

[2] Dante P. Martinelli and Ana Paula de Almeida, "Negotiation, Management, and Systems Thinking," *Systemic Practice and Action Research* 11, no. 3 (1998): 319–334, https://doi.org/10.1023/a:1022904331127.

[3] Roy J. Lewicki, Bruce Barry, and David M. Saunders, *Negotiation*, 7th ed. (New York, NY: McGraw-Hill Education, 2015).

[4] Dr Sunny Lee, "Negotiation: Tackling Our Misconceptions," *The Guardian*, October 6, 2021.

[5] "What Is Negotiation? Definition of Negotiation, Negotiation Meaning," *The Economic Times*, n.d.

[6] Jonathan Moules, "Negotiation Skills Prove Their Real-World Worth," *Financial Times*, March 1, 2021.

[7] Ashira Prossack, "The Benefits of Everyday Negotiations," *Forbes*, February 13, 2018.

"By failing to prepare,
 you are preparing to fail."

—BENJAMIN FRANKLIN

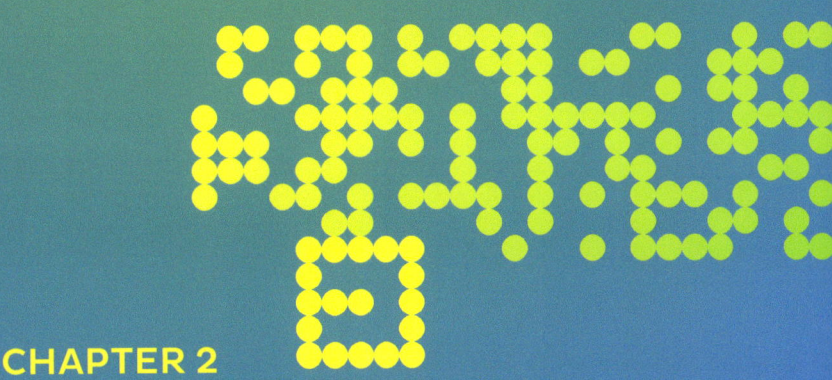

CHAPTER 2

THE NEGOTIATION PROCESS: PREPARING, ACTING, AND REVIEWING

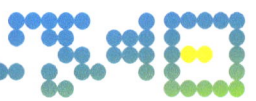

HOW IT WORKS

This chapter focuses on the negotiation process, which unfolds in three key stages: preparing, acting, and reviewing. The structure of the chapter reflects this progression, with each section dedicated to one of these phases. In the following pages, crucial topics are explored, including profiles of the parties, the mandate, sources of negotiating power, dynamics of the negotiation, and the vital function of the post-negotiation review. You'll be doing a variety of activities to cover this material, including reading and working on dynamic tasks (survey questions, video interviews, and your diary). Below, you'll find detailed instructions on how to engage with this chapter of the book.

2.1 PREPARING

The first part of the chapter is about preparation, which amounts to laying the foundation for the rest of the negotiation process. First, we'll talk about the relevance of profiling – this means yourself and the other party. You'll also learn where to search for information to prepare for negotiations, and what sources allow you to get a variety of input. Finally, you'll find out about the most popular negotiation styles, and how to adjust your own style to the relative context.

SELF-ASSESSMENT
Discover your negotiation orientation profile through a self-assessment survey.

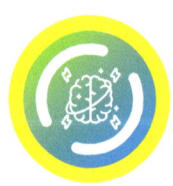

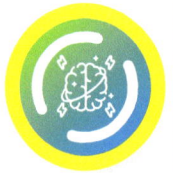

SELF-ASSESSMENT
We ask you to take the self-assessment to understand your negotiation style. Your responses will be included in the final chapter of the book.

2.2 ACTING

The second part of this chapter is about conducting the actual negotiation. You'll get insights on how to effectively do so, leveraging the previous preparation stage. This section also describes what team-based negotiation is and why it has its own specific dynamics, obstacles, and opportunities.

2.3 REVIEWING

After preparing and acting, the third stage of the negotiation process is reviewing the overall dynamics. In this section, we outline the necessary steps to assess the negotiation and better prepare for the next one.

VIDEO INTERVIEWS
Interviews with experts will enable you to see things from the perspectives of experienced practitioners from different countries, industries, and backgrounds.

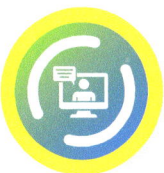

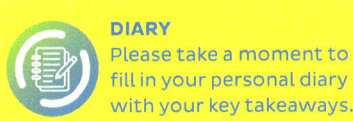

DIARY
Please take a moment to fill in your personal diary with your key takeaways.

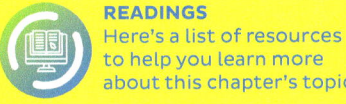

READINGS
Here's a list of resources to help you learn more about this chapter's topics.

SUMMARY

2.1 PREPARING

2.1.1 Profiling

A successful negotiation begins well before you enter the physical or virtual room and sit down at the table with another party. Effective negotiation processes are structured into three stages: preparing, acting, and reviewing. In this section, we'll examine the first one.

In preparing for a negotiation, it's beneficial to start by assessing your own negotiation orientation profile. This reflects your personal characteristics, preferences, and tendencies, and helps determine how to approach and participate in negotiations. The negotiation orientation is influenced by the mandate (see section 2.1.2), so it's important to know your own orientation to see how well it aligns with this mandate. Several factors contribute to your negotiation orientation profile, but here we'll give just a few examples of the constituent elements.

The first is how you like to approach the different stages of the negotiation process. For instance, when we talk about the opening phase, you might prefer to introduce the subject of the negotiation, or focus on building rapport during the initial part of the meeting, or listen carefully to the other party to gather more information, or try to be the first to make a proposal.

Moreover, it's essential to understand your aspirations and underlying attitudes toward the process. For example, do you expect to win every negotiating situation? Are you afraid of disrupting the negotiation? Do you tend to focus more on the other party rather than the object of the negotiation? Are you inclined to call in experts who handle the negotiation on your behalf? Do you ask for breaks during the negotiation, or do you allow the other party to take breaks?

Reflecting on your negotiation orientation also involves considering the challenges that are most critical for you. For example, is negotiating under pressure, with a deadline, particularly difficult for you? Do you struggle when the mandate is unclear? Is it challenging when the parties lack the necessary technical competencies to have a meaningful discussion? Do you find it difficult to maintain an effective balance between the rational and relational dimensions of the negotiation? Are you concerned about not having an actionable alternative in case the current negotiation fails? Or perhaps you feel you're at a disadvantage when you don't know the other side well enough?

These questions help identify your negotiation preferences and your general approach, which influence how you navigate the overall process and interact with others.

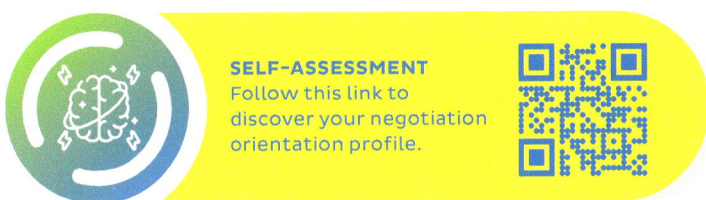

SELF-ASSESSMENT
Follow this link to discover your negotiation orientation profile.

Data collection and analysis are crucial to understanding the negotiation orientation profile of other parties. So being well-informed lays the groundwork for successful negotiations and helps avoid critical missteps.

Information can be obtained from open sources (e.g., articles, personal web pages, public speeches at conferences, forums, and workshops), which may provide a great deal of useful input on other negotiators as well as on the organization they represent (such as the corporate strategy, key partners, flagship projects, priorities, relations with the authorities, innovations initiatives, and financial reports). Furthermore, reviewing public interviews by each party (remember, yourself included) can offer deeper understanding by allowing you to observe not only the content of their responses but also their unique style of communication – how they speak, handle questions, and express themselves. (See Chapter 5 on communication.) If negotiators have authored a book, it's wise to read it, not only to gather valuable insights but also to strengthen communication and demonstrate that you value their work.

Information via networking can also prove invaluable. By leveraging professional networks or engaging with a company's partners, you can gain crucial intelligence on each party's negotiation profile. In this regard, the power of big data cannot be overlooked; collecting data from social media platforms can be a major asset when negotiating.

You can also gather constructive information during the negotiation itself, for instance, by inviting the other party to introduce themselves at the beginning of the meeting and listening carefully to their presentation. This can reveal insights about the other party's organization, the dynamics within their negotiation team (if applicable), and their personal characteristics, negotiation style, and emotional tendencies.

Other than negotiators and organizations, you should also research the sector and the broader domain. This is particularly crucial when negotiating with organizations outside your field, where your expertise may be more limited. So, you need to understand the general context, trends, key players, major events, and pertinent legislation.

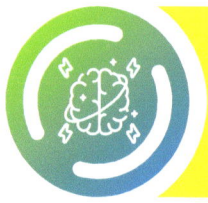

SELF-ASSESSMENT
Before reading about negotiation styles, we suggest you take a self-assessment of your own style. The following section presents each style and explains its relative advantages and disadvantages.

Preferred negotiation styles

Negotiation styles refer to "personal preference for how to negotiate," in other words, how you would prefer to engage in discussions and make decisions. Be aware that when negotiating on behalf of an organization, your preferences may not align with the organization's mandate, that is, what the organization expects you to achieve. (See the next section.) In any case, understanding your style helps you prepare more effectively for negotiations, as it allows you to recognize the gap between "how I would like to negotiate" (negotiation style) and "how I should negotiate," (again, as dictated by your mandate).

Based on the previous online activity, you are now aware of your own preferred negotiation style(s). Below we discuss each one, highlighting pros and cons in the context of a negotiation.

1. Negotiators with a *competitive style* tend to take a win-lose attitude. This can be suitable in a situation when they're asked to maximize the outcome from a short-term perspective. (See Chapter 3 on negotiation strategies.) It can also be appropriate to respond to the other party's tough, adversarial style, at least until they change their strategy and become more collaborative. On the downside, a competitive style can lead to conflict and even ruin the relationship between the parties.

2. A *collaborative style* generally means a preference to look for a win-win situation. This can prove to be effective when there is a shared level of trust between negotiators, and their goal is to achieve mutual satisfaction, as far as possible. One of the main disadvantages of a collaborative style is time management; the negotiation process may take up excessive time and energy. Moreover, negotiators acting according to their preferred collaborative style need to be ready to deal with potential opportunistic behaviors from the other side. In this regard, reciprocal trust can reduce the probability of getting caught up in a similar dynamic.
3. Negotiators with a *compromising style* prefer to get at least something out of the negotiation, but they are willing to make concessions to the other party. In other words, their reasoning goes like this: "I lose something and win something, and so does the other side." When adopting this style, negotiators stop halfway to achieving satisfactory goals. Such an approach is beneficial when negotiators enjoy similar status and negotiating power, or when negotiators can quickly find a solution that satisfies all parties (which saves time). If you use a compromising style, you need to clearly set priorities and determine what's most important to you, and what you're willing to sacrifice to achieve the compromise. There are some disadvantages here, such as the risk that critical or strategic matters may not be given adequate weight. Additionally, with a compromising style, neither party fully achieves their objectives.
4. An *avoidance style* emerges as a preference to sidestep conflictual situations instead of facing them. This can be dependent on various factors, such as low interest, unwillingness to be involved in a dispute, and emotional discomfort during a negotiation. In this case, negotiators tend to postpone any serious discussions, which can be useful to de-escalate conflicts or tensions among the parties. By the same token, sometimes postponing can be used as a technique (not as part of a negotiation style). In fact, avoiding negotiations is a way to put pressure on the other side, to prompt them to offer concessions or make the first move. This may have some possible disadvantages of procrastination which can become worse over time. When the other side employs an avoidance style, the best response is to encourage open dialogue, try to build trust, and emphasize the importance of reaching a solution rather than stalling or avoiding discussions altogether.

5. Negotiators with an *accommodating style* tend to be more willing to make concessions than to extract value from the other party. You may find this style is effective when the outcome of the negotiation is less important for you than it is for the other party. Here the model that applies is, "I give, the other side takes." The reason for using such a strategy may be the realization that a concession now will bring benefits in the future. A response when the other party adopts an accommodating style may be to first express gratitude for the fact that your interests are highly valued. At the same time, it is equally crucial not to accept all the concessions you're offered, as this can weaken the long-term relationship. An accommodating style has some possible disadvantages; it can reduce the capacity to influence the other side, and the negotiator's long-term credibility.

2.1.2 Defining the right mandate

Equally relevant to the negotiation orientation and preferred style, is the mandate from the organization in question. This defines the framework within which the negotiator is empowered to make decisions and specifies the conditions under which agreements can be reached. In general, the mandate delineates the negotiator's decision-making authority and must be drawn up with the participation of the stakeholders that the negotiator represents.

When drafting a mandate, it is vital to clearly detail the purpose of the negotiation, the desired and undesired outcomes, the type of relationship to create with the other party, priorities, the level of decision-making, and available resources. These would include material, financial, administrative resources, e.g., salient information, co-branding, quality level, price, salary, quantity, delivery schedule, and project budget. Decision-making necessitates an understanding of the boundaries of the negotiator's autonomy. For example, when negotiating a price, there are limits to the range within which negotiators have the right to make decisions themselves. Furthermore, being aware of constraints is equally critical (such as the level of information about the reasons behind each resource to be negotiated, budgetary restrictions, deadlines, or other conditions).

An often overlooked but vital element of a mandate is the alignment of diverse stakeholders' interests. For example, let's say that the department for international markets of Company A is preparing for a negotiation with international Partner B. Several resources including the long-term relationship, the product quality, the price, and the market share to be achieved will be discussed. Although Company A is represented by its department, several other stakeholders in the same company may be interested in that negotiation. Therefore, when compiling the mandate, it's essential to map out all the stakeholders and their interests in the negotiation. Moreover, a transparent system of communication with all concerned parties is especially important when there are unexpected developments where their input may be critical in recalibrating the negotiation strategy.

In general, well-defined mandates make successful negotiations possible, mitigating the risk of internal conflicts (between different departments in the organization, for example). Such mandates also create a positive image of the organization, demonstrating to the other side that there is a high level of alignment between negotiators and their stakeholders.

2.1.3 Drawing up a negotiation storyboard

The negotiation storyboard can be compared to a film script; it outlines the general idea and the plotline, assigning roles to the cast and describing how they should prepare. But unlike a film script, the plot development is not predetermined. Instead, negotiators need to map out all the possible scenarios, like in a chess game or on a decision tree.

A decision tree is a useful concept and a tool frequently employed in decision-making processes. Essentially, it consists of an analytical framework that allows us to evaluate various scenarios and the corresponding actions and responses we might take in each one.

To better understand this, consider the analogy of a chess game once again, where we think about what a player can do with a pawn or a knight, for example, and then we consider what we would do if our opponent moves with one of those pieces. The same mechanics apply when making decisions in negotiations. If the other party offers us a lower price, for instance, we may offer fewer resources; if they offer us a higher price, we may agree with the level of resources we originally proposed. In general, the idea of the decision tree approach is that we develop not isolated solutions, or a sequence of solutions, but a system of decisions, which includes analyses of a variety of possible developments and our responses to each one. In this vein, a decision tree empowers systematic thinking, helping us navigate complex decisions by mapping out potential choices. When developing a negotiation storyboard, it is useful to draw up a decision tree in the form of questions or suggestions, arguments or proposals that the other side can make, and how we can answer them.

A negotiation storyboard is an important tool, and much of the negotiation depends on how well it's prepared and the level of detail. It's vital to define the main objective of the negotiation and the expected outcome. Since negotiations, in particular collaborative negotiations, can often be complex (in terms of number of resources, objectives, and outcomes) it is reasonable to describe in the negotiation agenda the priorities in achieving the objectives for each resource.

2.1.4 Sources of negotiating power and knowing how and when to use them

Negotiating power is the ability of a party to influence the process and outcome of negotiations based on available sources. There are several such sources, however it is generally recognized that the three that carry the most weight are information, time and alternatives (in particular, the BATNA – the best alternative to a negotiated agreement).

1. Unquestionably, *information* is the most relevant source of negotiating power. Having access to the negotiation orientation profile of each party, along with other critical information, can notably impact the course of discussions. This could include a key insight into an ongoing deal, knowledge of an upcoming invention, or plans to launch a new product that could reshape the entire market. While such high-stakes information is rare, other types, like a strong understanding of market conditions and emerging trends, can also offer an appreciable advantage.
2. *Time* can create a certain amount of pressure, including psychological pressure. When a decision has to be made quickly, negotiators are inclined to make concessions, and to refuse to take a break; they may also agree to less favorable terms if they are under stress. For example, you can offer to fulfill a given order much faster but for a higher price; if the other party is acting under time constraints, then they may be willing to accept such a proposal.
3. The third source of negotiating power is represented by *alternatives* to a negotiation, and in particular the best alternative or BATNA. A clearly,

professionally formulated BATNA can be a persuasive argument in negotiations. Knowing exactly what you would do if there is no agreement with the other party, you gain confidence in moving toward the desired goals. (See Chapter 3 for a detailed discussion on alternatives and BATNA.)

4. Another key source of power is *expertise*. Demonstrating unique or high-level expertise can strengthen your arguments considerably. For instance, having a skilled expert on your side who proposes a specialized technical solution can give you a distinct advantage in negotiations.
5. *Networking* also acts as a source of power, for example, when you can go to an influential person in the field and get their support and a recommendation. Sometimes simply knowing influential people can carry considerable weight. For example, in case of a high level of perceived uncertainty (like in the process of digital transformation) change agents in an organization, who would also be effective negotiators, may call on influential people with high social status or standing to reduce the uncertainty as perceived by their colleagues. In this way they would alleviate their individual resistance to change in their organization.
6. *Reputation and brand* are two other significant sources of power. Obviously, a strong brand opens many doors in negotiations. Reputation can be both at the level of the company (referring to company values, high quality products and services, ranking in its market of reference) or the negotiator (having a successful track record in previous deals, being known to keep their promises). When sitting at the table with a highly reputable negotiator, the other party may be more inclined to make concessions, or might be open to accepting the proposed terms and conditions, anticipating that collaboration will enhance their own reputation. This could also lead to strengthening the company's market position and gaining access to high-profile partners, creating additional strategic advantages for both sides.
7. *Personal qualities* are also a strong source of power, e.g., charisma, friendliness, humor, and charm.
8. Nowadays, *creativity and innovation* are more and more valued in negotiation. Both can help generate alternatives, in turn enhancing the likelihood of finding shared agreement that more fully satisfies each party.
9. Understanding the *culture* of all the negotiators, as well as the traditions, values and communication peculiarities of the other party, is also a vital

source of negotiating power. (See Chapter 6 for a deep discussion on culture in negotiation.) Finally, knowing some other general information like films, writers, and great figures from the other party's country can also have a positive impact on the course of negotiation.

2.2 ACTING

2.2.1 Managing the meeting

A critical aspect of effective negotiations is the meeting itself, including how exactly to choose the venue, how to prepare the physical or virtual room (see Chapter 5 on communication), and how to structure the dynamics of the negotiations.

Taking care of seemingly small issues can also play a big role in determining the outcome. For example, an apparently insignificant nuance (such as calling for a break) can have a relevant impact on the course of negotiations. If the meeting becomes heated and emotions get out of control, a break is an effective way to bring the negotiations back to a constructive, calmer climate. (Refer to Chapter 3 for a case study on the importance of breaks and see Chapter 4 on emotions.)

If we plan to conduct negotiations in a collaborative manner, a salient aspect is to create the appropriate atmosphere where all parties feel comfortable making comments and asking questions. There are many techniques that can be applied to do this, from choosing a comfortable place for negotiations, dealing with emotions, and using proper negotiation techniques (see Chapter 3). All this is very helpful in finding more flexible solutions.

As a general rule, having a clear structure for negotiations is an effective way to create a positive atmosphere and a comfortable environment. When the schedule is set and all parties understand the agenda, the level of uncertainty decreases, leading to a greater sense of calm and comfort for everyone involved.

Successful negotiations require a balanced approach, combining thorough preparation, flexibility, and transparent communication. Moreover, this allows you to cope with unexpected turns in negotiations and to adapt quickly to changing circumstances.

2.2.2 Team-based vs individual negotiators

Negotiations can be conducted individually or in a team. The peculiarity of individual negotiations is that a single person assumes all responsibility, including decision-making, establishing and modifying the strategy of negotiations, and achieving the negotiation outcomes. In this situation, the negotiator can tailor the process to align with personal strengths and preferences, while keeping in mind the mandate in question. By the same token, individual negotiation requires a major effort, as all aspects of preparation are taken on by a single person. This includes gathering information, formulating the strategy, and running the meetings.

Although an experienced, self-confident negotiator can approach negotiations individually, depending on the complexity of the issues on the table, working as a team can also offer many advantages. A negotiation team is a group of people who are selected to represent the joint interests of an organization; they negotiate by leveraging their strengths, knowledge, and perspectives. Team-based negotiations have specific dynamics, obstacles, and opportunities.

Usually, the team's structure and composition are determined by several factors, for example, each team member can represent a different area of expertise (e.g., people and culture, operations, supply chain, marketing, software, finance, or product design or technical features). Forming a negotiation team can also serve as a strategic move to showcase members who are highly skilled experts. In addition, a team of negotiators is better able to scan the situation more accurately from different points of view. For instance, perhaps one team member is more experienced in assessing the emotions conveyed by tone of voice and body language; another is more focused on the substance and facts pertinent to the negotiations.

Team-based negotiations, to be successful, have their own specific requirements. For example, it's crucial to prepare and profile each team member. What's more, everyone must have a clear understanding of what the goal is, what aspects are useful to emphasize, and what shouldn't be mentioned at all.

It's also critical to clearly assign roles within the team, ensuring that everyone involved knows their specific responsibilities and even the sequence in which they will intervene. For instance, before beginning, the team should decide who will make the introductions, who will make the opening remarks, and who will address each specific topic. Without proper coordination, issues can arise. For example, if the lead negotiator gives an opening statement and unexpectedly hands over the discussion of technical details to another team member, this can create confusion and disrupt the flow of the negotiation. Thorough preparation and clear role assignments prevent such missteps, ensuring a smooth, cohesive presentation.

So as mentioned above, the team should hold at least one meeting prior to the negotiations to thoroughly discuss and agree on the position of the team, the interests and goals of the negotiations, and the responsibility and role of each team member. Effective, well-organized communication within the team is essential to avoid sending conflicting signals during the negotiation. If team members insist on contrasting arguments during negotiations, it can create a feeling that the negotiation team isn't clear about their goal, or worse still, that their statements are not true. So the team should demonstrate full agreement, mutual support, and good relations among its members. And if there are internal conflicts between team members, it's essential to evaluate whether they can work effectively together without allowing tensions to surface.

When negotiating as a team, which is particularly relevant in collaborative contexts, some roles can be assigned during storyboard preparation. Each member of the negotiation team takes on a specific task, contributing to the overall success of the negotiation. Below the six typical roles are presented.

The *lead negotiator*, who holds primary responsibility for the outcome, is often given considerable authority and oversees the entire negotiation process. This includes managing the negotiation team, formalizing major decisions, assigning roles, and guiding the strategy throughout the discussion.

The *primary negotiator* is the main point of contact with the other party. While this individual may have less authority than the leader, they are essential in building rapport and maintaining clear communication. Their key role is to gather information and, at the appropriate moment, facilitate problem-solving to reach an agreement. The same person can play the part of both lead and primary negotiator.

The *critic* plays a crucial role in preparing for the negotiation by identifying weaknesses in the arguments and the strategy. This team member searches for flaws in reasoning, anticipates possible objections, and ensures that the team's approach is as airtight as possible.

The *relater* or *bridge builder* is responsible for creating a positive atmosphere and establishing strong interpersonal connections. They handle any distractions, preserve a constructive environment, and ensure the negotiation remains calm and focused, intervening to defuse tensions or de-escalate critical situations. Their role is to foster a collaborative spirit and prevent the discussions from becoming confrontational.

The *situation board representative* captures key points and information on a whiteboard, a digital board, or a flip chart, for the entire team to see. This allows everyone to stay on the same page and refer back to essential details as the negotiation progresses.

The *specialist* contributes specific knowledge relevant to the technical aspects of the negotiation. For example, in negotiations regarding car deliveries, a logistics expert is needed who will be familiar with all the nuances and peculiarities of this service, and clearly state technical requirements.

Each of these team members should ensure that the negotiation process is comprehensive and carefully prepared.

2.3 REVIEWING

2.3.1 Once a final decision is made

After each negotiation, a reflection session is extremely useful. This involves reviewing the dynamics that emerged throughout the process to highlight key insights and lessons learned that can inform future negotiations. When reviewing the negotiation, there are several dimensions to consider.

1. *Goals:* Have you achieved the expected goals? If not, why? What can you do better next time? Were these goals articulated with clarity and constructiveness? How can you define them more clearly?
2. *Mandate:* Did you ask for changes/adjustments to the mandate during the negotiations? Did you need to adapt your negotiation style given the mandate in question? If so, how did you do so?
3. *Strategy:* Did you switch your strategy? If so, why? How did it happen? Did you and the other side adopt the same strategy? What could you have done to get the other party to adopt the same strategy as yours?
4. *Negotiating parties:* How did each negotiator behave? Did this influence your behavior? If so, how? What behaviors by the other party did you approve of? Which ones did you not appreciate? Was the profiling (of

yourself and other side) effective enough? If not, how can you improve it? This analysis should encompass not only the direct participants but also the behind-the-scenes influencers who may impact the negotiation process and outcomes.
5. *Sources of power:* What sources of power did you leverage? What about the other side? Did all the negotiators use their sources of power effectively? If not, how can everyone do better?
6. *Negotiation styles:* It's helpful to analyze the negotiation styles employed by you and the other party, including strengths and weaknesses. How can you better align your negotiation style with your mandate and the negotiation situation?
7. *Communication style:* What style did you adopt? How about the other party? Did you notice any change in communication styles? If so, why? What are your strengths? And the other side's strengths? How can you improve your communication style?
8. *Information:* Did you collect complete, useful information for the negotiation? If not, what was missing? Did any new information come up during the negotiation? How could you improve your information management?
9. *Strengths and weaknesses, areas for improvement:* What is one of your strengths? How can you use it in the next negotiation? What are your weaknesses and how can they be improved? Highlight areas for personal growth, such as enhancing emotional stability or mastering advanced communication techniques, to refine your approach in future negotiations.
10. *Outcomes:* Did you sign an agreement? Under what terms? Are you fully satisfied with the results of the negotiation? If not, why? What would you do differently to improve next time?

All these steps will allow you to compile a repository of data about the negotiation. What's more, this will help you to conduct successful negotiations with the same party if the opportunity arises and enable you to better manage negotiations in general in the future.

In the next chapter, we'll examine the main negotiation strategies, how to apply them, and how to define the negotiation space.

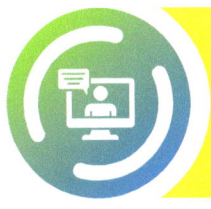

VIDEO INTERVIEWS
We ask experts the best way to profile the parties in a negotiation, how to deal with unexpected circumstances that might arise, and more.

DIARY
Please take a moment to fill in your personal diary with your key takeaways.

READINGS
Here's a list of resources to help you learn more about this chapter's topics.

SUMMARY

NEGOTIATION PROFILE	Unique set of characteristics, preferences, and tendencies that define how you approach and participate in negotiations, to include negotiation orientation profile and preferred style
RESOURCES	Material goods, financial assets, and intangible assets you are authorized to exchange during the negotiation
STYLES	Preferences on how to engage in discussions, make decisions, and navigate the process: • competitive • collaborative • compromising • avoidance • accommodating
MANDATE	Sets out the framework within which the negotiator is empowered to make decisions, and specifies the conditions under which agreements can be reached
STORYBOARD	Describes the general idea, the storyline, assigns roles, and describes how to prepare
NEGOTIATING POWER	The ability of a party to influence the process and the outcome of negotiations

39

TEAM-BASED NEGOTIATION	Roles in a negotiation team: • lead negotiator • primary negotiator • critic • relater or bridge builder • situation board representative • expert or technical specialist
REVIEWING	Key dimensions: • goals • mandate • strategy • parties • sources of power • negotiation styles • communication style • information • strengths and weaknesses, areas for improvement • outcomes

"There is no favorable wind for the sailor who doesn't know where to go."

_SENECA

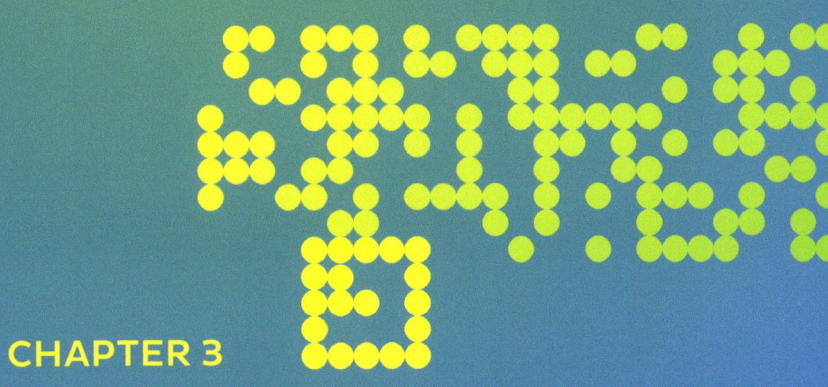

CHAPTER 3

NEGOTIATION STRATEGIES AND TECHNIQUES

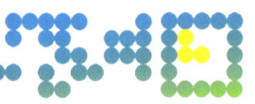

HOW IT WORKS

This chapter addresses the main negotiation strategies and their key differences; you'll also learn about the related topics of BATNA, WATNA and ZOPA. To conclude, case studies illustrate negotiations in different contexts. You'll be doing a series of activities, such as reading, answering survey questions, watching video interviews, and writing in your diary. Below, you'll find detailed instructions on how to engage with this chapter of the book.

SURVEY
To start this chapter, you'll answer questions to get you thinking about negotiation strategies.

3.1 DETERMINING THE APPROPRIATE STRATEGY AND TECHNIQUES

In this section, you'll learn about the main strategies of negotiation, their features and relative techniques.

3.2 ALTERNATIVES AND ZOPA

Here you'll find out about alternatives (BATNA, WATNA) and common ground in the negotiation space (ZOPA).

SELF-REFLECTION QUESTIONS
Here you'll be asked to think about first distributive and then integrative strategies in negotiations.

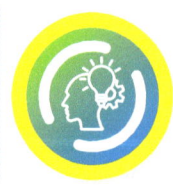

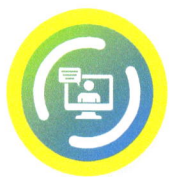

VIDEO INTERVIEWS
Now you can watch the video interviews to hear experts' perspective.

CHAPTER 3 | NEGOTIATION STRATEGIES AND TECHNIQUES

3.3 SWITCH FROM DISTRIBUTIVE TO INTEGRATIVE

In this section, you'll discover the primary reasons for choosing a negotiation strategy and what factors drive the transition from a distributive to an integrative strategy.

3.4 SHORT CASES

Included here are some cases illustrating the transition from distributive to integrative strategy and the reasons behind it, such as emotional reactions, cultural aspect, third party influence, and economic factors.

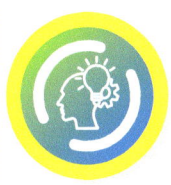

SELF-REFLECTION QUESTIONS
At this point, you'll be asked to think about the transition from a distributive to an integrative strategy.

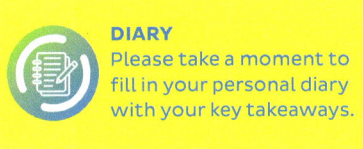

DIARY
Please take a moment to fill in your personal diary with your key takeaways.

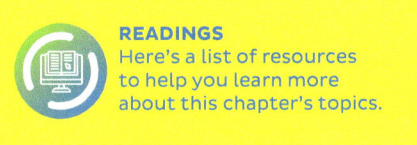

READINGS
Here's a list of resources to help you learn more about this chapter's topics.

SUMMARY

43

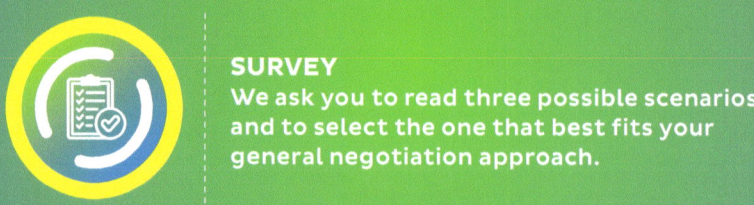

SURVEY
We ask you to read three possible scenarios and to select the one that best fits your general negotiation approach.

3.1 DETERMINING THE APPROPRIATE STRATEGY AND TECHNIQUES

In any negotiation, whether it happens in the context of a business deal, B2B collaboration, a family situation, a cross-cultural scenario, or with internal discussions between company departments, strategies must be identified. There are two fundamental negotiation strategies: distributive (win-lose) and integrative (win-win).

With a *distributive* or *competitive strategy*, the negotiation is perceived as win-lose, or a zero-sum game, with only one side successfully reaching their goals. From this perspective, the goal of negotiations is to extract the greatest benefit, the best outcomes for yourself. Consequently, a distributive strategy is not aimed at building long-term relationships or future collaborations; instead, the focus is on short-term connections. That's why this strategy is also called a "position-based" negotiation. Moreover, usually distributive negotiations mainly involve a very limited number of resources, with a predetermined range of values that will not change (hence the expression "fixed pie"). A low level of information sharing is a typical of this strategy.

The distributive strategy is divided into two subtypes: attacking and defending. The first involves quite aggressive behavior, harsh conditions, ultimatums, and even threats on a professional level. Defensive strategies in contrast consist of non-combative statements and a more diplomatic tone. The approach is to explain the reasons for proposing a certain solution, with the aim of influencing or persuading the other party to achieve your goal.

A distributive strategy can be adopted in situations where you have no interest in further collaborations with the other party, or when you have far greater bargaining power (for instance, more time, more information about the situation than the other party, more resources, or if you have a monopoly).

When dealing with the other side's competitive strategy, it's essential to remain calm, prepare well-supported arguments, and present counterproposals. No matter the competitive strategy you adopt, the future is uncertain, and you may need to negotiate with the same party or someone connected to them on some other occasion. Consequently, you might want to adopt a collaborative strategy (and encourage the other party to do the same) by demonstrating its benefits, such as fostering a cooperative environment and achieving better outcomes for both parties.

With a distributive strategy, the atmosphere of the negotiations is often tense and demanding, creating a high-pressure environment. Such a context can contribute to the emotional instability of the negotiators. (See Chapter 4 about the role of emotions in negotiation.) In fact, if you don't keep your emotions in check, this can undermine your effectiveness, leading you to make mistakes and ultimately accept undesirable outcomes. In this setting, managing your emotions is crucial.

The opposite of a distributive strategy is an *integrative* or *collaborative strategy*. The objective here is to respect the interests of everyone in finding a win-win outcome, a joint creative decision that brings benefits to all parties. That's why creative problem-solving serves as a key skill. Integrative negotiation is forward-facing, focused on long-term relationships and partnerships, exploring potential opportunities of working together in the future. A large set of resources and relative values (useful for "expanding the pie") can be very effective in achieving this goal. The collaborative nature of this strategy stimulates a high level of information sharing between parties.

Other than openness and creativity, which we've already mentioned, trust is the third key characteristic of the integrative strategy. In an integrative negotiation the atmosphere is rather calm; the parties carefully listen to one another, finding common ground with the aim of making decisions that are favorable to all. Also, from the point of view of managing emotions, integrative negotiations are more amicable and relaxed than distributive ones.

A range of *techniques* are used with the two different strategies. Within the framework of distributive strategy, some classic techniques are:

- *Time pressure*, which means setting a deadline and explaining that it's necessary to make a decision within a certain period. (For instance, there's an urgent deadline for participating in a tender.)

- *The use of silence* can be extremely helpful; indeed, silence should not be feared. In a theater performance, an artistic pause is considered a powerful means of expression; the same is true in negotiations. Pausing is an effective way to get more information, prompting the other party to fill the silence and possibly make a new proposal.
- *Good cop/bad cop* is where one negotiator is more hard line, and the other offers more flexible terms and milder manners.
- *"My hands are tied"* equates to claiming that, unfortunately, we can't offer any more because we don't have the power, or external circumstances don't allow us to change the terms.
- *Tactical concessions* consist of one party giving a little ground to make bigger gains from the other party.
- *Destabilizing* involves using various tools to apply pressure on the other party, creating feelings of discomfort and anxiety. When that party experiences such unease, they will be more likely to make mistakes and concessions.

With the integrative strategy, the suggested technique is to follow a three-step process. At the heart of this strategy is active listening, essential not only to demonstrate interest in the other negotiating party but also to help you gather valuable insights and build rapport and trust. The three steps are as follows:

1. *Handshaking:* Establishing a connection with the other party.
2. *Structuring:* Defining the rules of the negotiation, e.g., deciding beforehand how to arrange the meetings, when to ask a third party to join as a mediator, how to discuss the resources of the negotiation (one by one or as a package).
3. *Acting:* Conducting the negotiation following the structure.

Whatever the strategy and techniques adopted, it's vital to develop a response behavior schema, for instance, in the format of a decision tree. (If Party A says X, then I can respond with Y or Z.)

Usually negotiations are not dichotomous, either fully distributive or integrative. Actually, negotiations often employ both strategies. In other words, during the negotiation process, one or both parties may switch from one strategy to the other. In many instances, negotiators might shift from a competitive to a collaborative strategy (and vice versa) depending on the specific circumstances at hand. This transition must be consistent with the mandate in question. If there is any doubt, negotiators have to first check with the party they're representing. Since unexpected behaviors and developments can happen, it's essential to remain flexible and open to adjusting your strategy if it enhances the negotiation outcome, within the framework of the given mandate.

3.2 ALTERNATIVES AND ZOPA

The process of negotiation is often highly complex; normally negotiators deal with a great deal of uncertainty. This means it's vital to be prepared for best and worst cases, and to figure out where the common ground may lie to find a possible solution.

BATNA (Best Alternative To a Negotiated Agreement) refers to the most favorable alternative that can be reached in a situation where Plan A (in a specific negotiation) will land on "no agreement." Defining BATNA in advance is a crucial move, since it allows you to set the boundaries beyond which you will walk away from a deal, since it does not meet your requirements. It's important to highlight the distinction between BATNA and the walk-away point. The latter is the minimum outcome you would accept before leaving the negotiation, while the BATNA is the best option available if the negotiation fails.

A great way to understand the concepts of BATNA and the walk-away point is through the following example. Let's say you're negotiating with an international supplier (A) for the procurement of a specific technological component. You've been authorized to pay a unit price ranging between €10 and €12 (among the other resources to be negotiated). You've already investigated alternative offers from other international suppliers for the same component and currently have these in hand: Partner B offers a unit price of €13; Partner C, €12; and Partner D, €11.50. If your negotiation with Partner A lands on "no agreement," and assuming your interest is only the price, then your best alternative is to go with the offer from Partner D. Based on your mandate, you've set your walk-away value, which is not necessarily same of your BATNA. Going back to the previous example, while your BATNA unit price is €11.50, let's assume (given your mandate) you have a walk-away unit price value of €12.50. The walk-away represents the value that you are willing to accept in a negotiation; beyond this value (lower or higher, depending on your perspective), you are prepared to leave the table.

A three-step algorithm can be applied to determine your BATNA. The first step is to think through the actions you could take in case of unsuccessful negotiations; in other words, create a list of alternative solutions. The second step is to determine the value of each one considering not only material but also non-material benefits (e.g. reputational, long-term vs short-term perspective). Third, from all the possible alternatives, identify the one that works best for you.

Effective negotiators also work out their WATNA (Worst Alternative To a Negotiated Agreement). The WATNA refers to the least favorable outcome in a situation where the parties could not reach an agreement during negotiations. Going back to the previous example, again your primary intention is to negotiate with Partner A. In case the conclusion of this negotiation is "no agreement," your worst alternative is to go with Partner B (who offers a unit price of €13). Identifying both BATNA and WATNA helps to anticipate the direction of a negotiation, and at the same time it increases your negotiating power. (In Chapter 2, see the section on negotiating power.)

It's also essential to delineate the Zone of Possible Agreement (ZOPA), the range within which all parties can find mutually acceptable solutions. In essence, the ZOPA represents the intersection between the minimum and maximum limits of the negotiating parties. Identifying this zone allows for a more focused negotiation process, ensuring efforts are directed towards outcomes that all sides can agree on. For example, let's say a company wants to negotiate the purchase of some office equipment; the company representative has been authorized to pay between €35,000 and €50,000, while the seller has permission to accept anywhere from €40,000 and €65,000. Consequently, the ZOPA is between €40,000 (minimum value of seller) and €50,000 (maximum budget of buyer). The two parties may not be initially open to sharing these figures with one another, so asking open-ended questions to better understand where the other party stands is a good technique.

To sum up, identifying BATNA, WATNA and ZOPA in advance is a crucial step to ensure a robust, well-defined framework and relevant expectations.

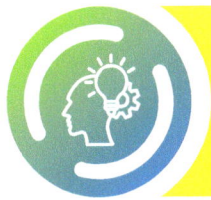

SELF-REFLECTION QUESTIONS
We ask you to describe two negotiation situations: one that was conducted using a distributive strategy and one using an integrative strategy.

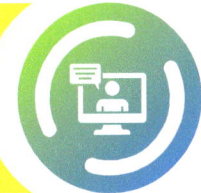

VIDEO INTERVIEWS
Now you can hear the experts describe their experience in this context, what they learned from it and how they changed their strategy, if they did.

3.3 SWITCH FROM DISTRIBUTIVE TO INTEGRATIVE

As mentioned, distributive and integrative strategies are not definitive or unchangeable. During negotiations, the participants may switch from one to another (if the mandate allows), a transition that can go in either direction and may be influenced by many factors. However, here we'll focus on the shift from distributive to integrative, as this represents a more constructive path.

Let's follow this example. Two parties start their negotiation applying a distributive strategy (centered on the result, to the detriment of long-term relations). But during the meetings, they receive some new information, or they come to understand certain things that were unclear before or were simply based on erroneous assumptions. As a result, they begin to see the potential benefits of long-term collaborations and future joint projects. In this scenario, the parties can switch from a distributive to an integrative strategy (if the mandate allows), where the focus is on problem-solving and finding win-win solutions.

The transition from one strategy to the other often occurs when the parties enter negotiations unaware of their shared goals and interests and then gradually come to recognize what they have in common during their discussion. As new information emerges, they see the value of collaborating, generating mutual benefits, and achieving common objectives through joint efforts. With this realization and the necessary mandate, the parties shift from a competitive stance to a cooperative one, embracing an integrative strategy.

Another driver for this shift may be the discovery of essential resources. Initially, one party might not know that the other possesses some critical assets, but during negotiations, this information may come to light. If these resources are useful to one or all the negotiators, they would find it both logical and advantageous to adopt a collaborative strategy.

Bringing a third party on board can facilitate the transition from a distributive to an integrative strategy, shifting the balance of power and transforming the negotiation dynamics. In this regard, in the next section you'll find two examples: one is the negotiation between two giants in the automotive industry, Fiat and Chrysler (Case 5); the second example is about an institutional negotiation (Case 4).

The mandate determines the strategy and defines the boundaries of your authority within the framework of the negotiation. Nevertheless, some factors may prompt you to switch negotiation strategy. (In this case, you need to check back with whoever gave you the mandate.) These are listed below.

- *Trust and openness:* When negotiations are built on these two aspects, there is an incentive to continue working together in the future.
- *Culture:* This factor influences the choice of strategy (see Chapter 6); in more competitive cultures, a distributive strategy is favored while in less competitive ones the opposite is true.
- *Bargaining power:* The negotiators with more (perceived or actual) power tend to dictate the strategy, and most often they opt for a distributive one.
- *Economic factors:* These also affect the choice of strategy, as shown in Case 5; sometimes even the economic power of a country has an impact on the way it approaches negotiations, especially at the level of national institutions.

Integrative negotiations occur more frequently than we can imagine. As a general – and crucial – recommendation, as we mentioned above, before deciding to go with a distributive strategy (even if required by your mandate), you should try to explore the possibility of exchanging a certain level of information and creating a long-term partnership.

In the next chapter, we will see how perceptions, biases, and emotions affect negotiations.

3.4 SHORT CASES

CASE 1 — A HIGH EMOTIONAL STATE MAKES IT DISTRIBUTIVE

The first case illustrates the transition from distributive to integrative strategy of a negotiation in a private setting, specifically a divorce. Initially, the spouses (Partner A and Partner B) each insist on getting all the property. This sounds like a perfect distributive strategy, i.e., the aim of the two is not cooperation or a future long-term relationship; they're each focusing exclusively on their own position. After a little reflection, they consider their children, and realize that they will have to continue communicating in the future. The partners take a step toward understanding each other's perspectives and begin discussing what matters most to them, identifying and addressing mutual interests. This marks a shift to an integrative negotiation strategy, a search for a compromise, where the focus lies on finding solutions that satisfy both parties' needs. Partner A will be travelling extensively on business; Partner B would like to spend as much time as possible with the children and is less inclined to change habits or move out of the family home. Both partners start looking for a creative solution they can both embrace. In the end, they decide that Partner B will stay in the apartment with the children while Partner A will retain ownership of the business, sharing a portion of the profits to ensure financial support for the children.

Ultimately, a deal is reached, and the priorities and wishes of all parties are respected. If the partners had continued to adhere to the distributive strategy, they would have faced a long trial, culminating in a less satisfactory agreement and negatively impacting the lives of all the family members.

CASE 2 — REDEFINING THE NEGOTIATION SPACE

Case 2 provides an example of expanding the negotiation space to facilitate the switch to an integrative strategy. This involves introducing new topics, issues, or dimensions into the negotiation, creating more space for dialogue and more opportunities for cooperation. A computer distribution firm is negotiating with a university, which wants to purchase a certain number of new devices for a computer lab. At the beginning, a distributive strategy is employed. The university demands a 10% discount, but the company states that no discount is possible.

The transition to an integrative strategy is done by expanding the negotiation space; in other words, by trying to increase the number of resources. The university representative asks if there are other ways to create shared value. In response,

the distributor offers options to extend the payment terms from one to three months. This decision is accepted by the university, since it can more effectively manage the cash flow and better allocate its budget for the next quarter.
By introducing new items on the agenda and broadening the scope of the discussion, both parties can find a more favorable outcome and create shared value.

CASE 3 — ADDING VALUE FOR THE OTHER PARTY

This case involves revealing details about your position, motivation, priorities, and limitations, encouraging the other party to share their own reasoning and insight, encouraging openness, and building rapport and trust. A company is hiring a marketing specialist. Initially, the negotiation follows a distributive strategy. The HR manager, Julia, is offering a starting salary of €3,000 (gross, per month), while the applicant Ivan demands €3,500 or he says he can't accept the job. Julia explains that the company is entering new markets and facing some financial constraints. After sharing this information, Julia then asks what would add value for Ivan beyond salary. He reveals that learning how to implement artificial intelligence in marketing is an important value for him. In response, Julia makes a new offer: the same €3,000 plus a high-level learning path on using AI in marketing. Ivan feels this new offer is fair, in line with his priorities, and consequently decides to accept it.
The exchange of information and the discussion of Ivan's motivations made the negotiation integrative, allowing both parties to better understand each other's interests and priorities and find a mutually beneficial solution.

CASE 4 — INSTITUTIONAL NEGOTIATION

This case is about the UNFCCC (UN Framework Convention on Climate Change) negotiations in Copenhagen on climate change in 2009. It serves as an excellent illustration of negotiation at the institutional level, where many factors come into play, specifically: economic power of various nations, the level of democracy, different cultures, pressure from interest groups and public opinion, resource utilization, and borrowed power from third parties.
The Copenhagen Climate Summit brought together the world's major countries to conclude a new agreement to replace the Kyoto Protocol. A series of negotiations were held under UNFCCC with more than 50 delegations from different countries discussing measures that would serve to halt climate change. The choice of distributive or integrative strategies was influenced by a number of factors:

- The economic power of the country represented by each institution is key. The greater the economic power of the country, the more likely the institution is to employ a distributive strategy, and vice-versa.
- The level of democracy also plays a role. The higher it is, the less likely institutions are to use a distributive strategy.
- The role of culture is also significant, as some cultures are more assertive and inclined toward distributive strategies, while others tend to favor collaborative strategy.
- Interest groups and public opinion have a voice. The stronger the pressure from such groups (e.g., business community, NGOs) and public opinion, the more institutions tend to adopt a distributive approach to negotiations.
- The power of a third party also comes into play. The case study shows how the inclusion of third parties (the press and researchers) may have influenced the change in strategy (if parties get a mandate for the transition), specifically prompting a shift from distributive to integrative.

Under the influence of the many factors outlined above, the negotiation did not take place on broad common ground, so it only lands on a political statement committing to limiting the global temperature rise to less than two degrees Celsius.

Source: Stefanie Bailer, "Strategy in the Climate Change Negotiations: Do Democracies Negotiate Differently?," *Climate Policy* 12, no. 5 (September 2012): 534–551.

CASE 5 — A THREE-PARTY NEGOTIATION

The negotiation between Fiat and Chrysler demonstrates the shift from a distributive to an integrative negotiation strategy between the two large automobile manufacturers, thanks to a third party. This case is interesting because it focuses on future collaboration and alliances. Initially the negotiation is between two parties, who adopt a distributive strategy. However, when the third party gets involved, the strategy switches from distributive to integrative.

As a starting point, Fiat (an Italian car company) had stable financial and market positions, and was seeking to introduce two lines (Alfa Romeo, Fiat 500) into the US market, Chrysler's home territory. In contrast, Chrysler, facing financial problems, was on the brink of bankruptcy. These two major companies engaged in negotiations to explore a potential collaboration and a global strategic alliance.

However, there were many tense moments. Chrysler needed financing, among other things, to meet the requirements of the US government, but Fiat was not willing to invest cash in the American company. At this point, the US government became involved as a third party, transforming the negotiations from bilateral to multilateral. The government decided to give Chrysler the necessary loan, but with the proviso that it had 30 days to conclude a deal with Fiat or face bankruptcy. In the end, Fiat and Chrysler successfully established a strategic alliance. Under the agreement, Chrysler received protection from its creditors, while Fiat secured a 20% stake in the partnership.

In general, compared to negotiations between two parties, multilateral negotiations stand apart, as they are more extensive and complex, involve a greater number of stakeholders, each with their own interests, and are more difficult to manage. However, having a large team of experts and stakeholders can have a positive effect; bringing an array of skills to the table makes it possible to highlight different perspectives as negotiations develop.

Fonte: Andrea Caputo, "Integrative Agreements in Multilateral Negotiations: The Case of Fiat and Chrysler", *International Journal of Business and Social Science* 3, no. 12 (June 2012): 167–180.

SELF-REFLECTION QUESTIONS
Go online and write up a negotiation scenario where your strategy was switching from distributive to integrative.

DIARY
Please take a moment to fill in your personal diary with your key takeaways.

READINGS
Here's a list of resources to help you learn more about this chapter's topics.

SUMMARY

DISTRIBUTIVE OR COMPETITIVE STRATEGY	• Low level of information sharing • Fixed pie • All parties are apparently satisfied • Focusing on short-term relationships • Focusing on your arguments
INTEGRATIVE OR COLLABORATIVE STRATEGY	• "Expanding the pie" • All parties are truly satisfied • Focusing on long-term relationships • Exploring other opportunities to work together • Problem-solving approach
TECHNIQUES FOR DISTRIBUTIVE STRATEGY	• Time pressure • Silence as a tactic • Good cop/bad cop • "My hands are tied" • Tactical concessions • Destabilization
3-STEP PROCESS FOR INTEGRATIVE STRATEGY	At the heart lies active listening and trust building. 1. Handshaking 2. Structuring 3. Acting
POSITION	What to get from the other party
INTERESTS	Sharing reasons underlying the requests of each side
BATNA	Best Alternative To a Negotiated Agreement – the most favorable solution that can be reached in a situation where Plan A will land on "no agreement"
WATNA	Worst Alternative To a Negotiated Agreement – the least favorable outcome in a situation where the parties cannot reach an agreement
ZOPA	Zone of Possible Agreement – the range within which all parties can find mutually acceptable solutions
TRANSITION FROM DISTRIBUTIVE TO INTEGRATIVE STRATEGY	Reasons the parties would transition: • They understand long-term relations, and the benefits of partnership and joint projects. • They discover common interests and goals. • They find resources that can be used jointly. • A third party may play an influential role. Factors driving this choice: • trust and openness • cultural dimension • bargaining power • economic factors

"If people define situations as real,
they are real in their consequences."
_WILLIAM ISAAC THOMAS
and DOROTHY SWAINE THOMAS

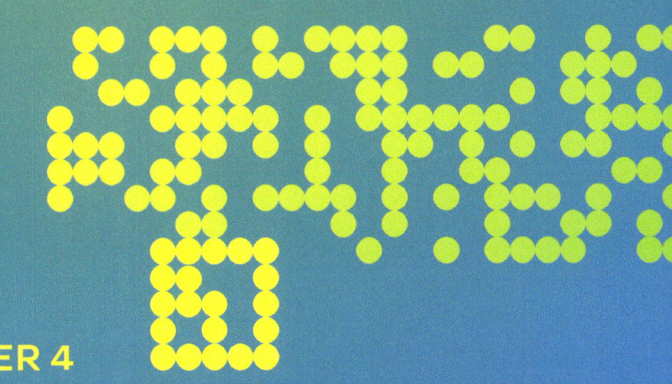

CHAPTER 4

PERCEPTIONS, BIASES, AND EMOTIONS

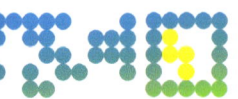

HOW IT WORKS

Negotiation is often erroneously viewed as a perfectly rational process, relying completely on cognitive abilities, analytical thinking, and logical decision-making. This chapter discusses how perceptions, biases, and emotions shape the process, adding depth to our understanding of what truly influences effective negotiations. You'll be reading the static sections and working on dynamic activities (survey questions, video interviews, and diary), with detailed instructions below on how to engage.

SURVEY
At the very beginning of this chapter, you'll be asked to think about the role of perceptions, biases, and emotions in negotiation by answering some questions.

4.1 MOST FREQUENT PERCEPTIONS AND BIASES

In this section, you'll learn how perceptions and biases influence negotiation, and how to overcome them.

4.2 EMOTIONS

In this section, we'll discuss which emotions most often arise in negotiations and how they can harm the process, the outcomes, and the long-term relationship with the other side. We'll also give you tips on how to work with your own emotions and the other party's.

CHAPTER 4 | PERCEPTIONS, BIASES, AND EMOTIONS

SURVEY
At the end of this chapter, you'll be asked to think again about how perceptions, biases, and emotions can affect negotiations.

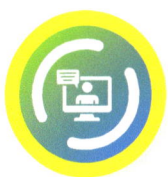

VIDEO INTERVIEWS
These interviews are an essential part of the book and are designed to offer you a practice-oriented outlook on negotiation.

DIARY
Please take a moment to fill in your personal diary with your key takeaways.

READINGS
Here's a list of resources to help you learn more about this chapter's topics.

SUMMARY

SURVEY
To what extent can perceptions and biases influence a negotiation process? And how meaningful are emotions when negotiating? Answer these and other self-reflection questions before continuing to read.

4.1 MOST FREQUENT PERCEPTIONS AND BIASES

Negotiation might appear to be a perfectly rational process. But in recent decades, the role of non-rational and non-cognitive factors has been capturing more and more attention. There are several reasons behind this. Human nature is not fully rational, operating as it does in two distinct systems: one rooted in intuition and instinct, and the other one in rational thinking. Added to this, negotiators often lack complete information and knowledge, so they may not have accurate decision-making criteria. Then there are perception errors that stop negotiators from arriving at the valid conclusions and making the right choices. What's more, there's a difference between facts and information and the way we perceive them. In fact, our perception is determined by our experience, values, cultural background, and social environment (among the other things).

Perception refers to how exactly we interpret information and influences negotiations through several mechanisms, for instance, shaping how each party evaluates the other's behaviors. As an example, a proposal might be seen as aggressive (even if it's not) simply because it's presented in an assertive manner. Perception also has a significant impact on building trust. Trustworthiness is a crucial factor in negotiation; when we perceive the other party as honest and reliable, we are more inclined to accept their idea or proposal.

Consider a negotiation between a local government and a large chain of shopping malls. The chain proposes building a shopping complex that addresses the needs of local residents (by creating community spaces and clubs, for instance), and supports local businesses by offering favorable conditions for local artisans (by charging lower rent for their workshops or stores). But the local government, which initially views the company as purely profit-driven, doesn't trust its intentions. The way to overcome this perception is through openness, demonstrating plans to incorporate the interests of the local community in the project.

Bias, in turn, can distort perceptions and influence the negotiators' processing abilities in terms of judgement, decision-making, and the overall negotiation. In other words, bias influences the way we perceive reality.

It is worth highlighting some of the most common biases. *Confirmation bias* occurs when a person focuses on information that confirms their initial assumptions and ignores data that support another point of view. In this case, the negotiator isn't trying to assess the situation objectively; instead, they're constantly searching for arguments that support their initial idea. This bias leaves room for both conscious and unconscious manipulation, adjustment, and distortion of the facts. As a result, the negotiator may miss opportunities to fully assess the situation, genuinely listen to the other party, adapt to new information, and remain flexible.

For example, during a first-time negotiation, the two parties don't trust each other yet. If one of them focuses on actions that confirm their initial belief, while ignoring new data or input from the other party, then this is very likely a case of confirmation bias. To overcome this, the key is to diligently analyze the whole stream of incoming information and try to consider what the other party is really saying and why.

Anchor bias occurs when a person relies on the first piece of information they receive, allowing it to shape their judgment regardless of subsequent facts. This type of bias is quite common. In fact, there's truth to the saying, "You never get a second chance to make a first impression," as that initial opinion can be remarkably hard to change. So, the anchor (the initial information) becomes an important starting point for negotiations, determining to a great extent the final decision.

Let's look at an example. Andrea intends to purchase a certain product. She reads an article on social media suggesting that the quality of the product she has identified is low. During the purchase negotiations, she is presented with certificates proving the quality of these same goods, yet she insists on a discount because of her perception of low quality. To overcome this bias, thoroughly collecting and analyzing all available information can be highly effective. (See Chapter 2.) When you have an extensive set of information (about the other party, the market dynamics, the quality of product or service, and the negotiator), then the first impression and the initial information won't hold so much sway, and you'll be able to make a more objective assessment.

Loss aversion bias can deeply influence decision-making processes. Losses often leave lasting marks on our memory. Research demonstrates that the distress and dissatisfaction caused by losses tend to be far more memorable than the joy of comparable victories. Often negotiators aim to avoid loss at any cost. But sometimes, like in a chess match, you have to give something to get something in return. With loss aversion bias, it's vital to remember that negotiators often tend to overestimate losses. So to overcome this tendency, you need to conduct a rational analysis of the negotiation and highlight the real value of the loss and gain; then outline a plan for what you can and cannot concede.

Overconfidence stands as one of the biggest biases, often disrupting rational judgment, impairing an objective assessment of situation, and influencing the quality of analysis and decision-making. This bias manifests in various ways: a false sense of control, an illusion of optimistic outcomes, and overestimation of negotiating skills, all of which can lead to adverse consequences. For example, when Tom is negotiating for a new job, he overestimates the value he can bring to his company and demands a salary and job title that would be impossible or illogical for his employer to offer. The company does not recognize the value that Tom insists on, which he believes would justify a much higher salary. The negotiation ends in a deadlock: Tom doesn't secure the new job, and the company has to continue the selection process. To mitigate the effects of overconfidence, it's advisable to prioritize thorough preparation, information gathering, and preliminary analysis, which help you see the objective picture and correctly assess the situation.

Status quo is a widespread bias, especially in cultures with extreme power distance. Status quo happens when a person with more authority or higher status is perceived as more influential or carrying more weight. This can clearly be a distortion of reality. For example, let's take Frank, a purchasing manager, and Joanne, a specialized, reputable market analyst. Frank is going to meet with Joanne to negotiate the purchase of a batch of Product A. Joanne claims that the market price for Product A is exactly what she initially proposed to Frank. Based on Joanne's status quo, Frank may be inclined to agree with Joanne just because he assumes she "knows exactly what the market price is for Product A."

To overcome the status quo bias, it's worth remembering that a person's elevated authority or status doesn't necessarily guarantee that they'll make strong arguments. Like in the previous case, to mitigate the effects of status quo, it's best to prioritize thorough preparation, information gathering, and preliminary analysis.

4.2 EMOTIONS

In the context of negotiations, it's essential to consider a comprehensive set of concrete factors, including economic conditions, the political environment, market trends, and competitive dynamics. In light of this, it's not surprising that for years the focus was placed on cognitive abilities, which facilitate gathering, processing, and analyzing relevant information, as well as formulating informed projections. This is why discussions around negotiations centered mainly on strategy and logic, overlooking other key components.

It was only a few decades ago that both researchers and practitioners began to recognize the significant role of emotions and emotional intelligence in negotiation. Even skilled negotiators experience a range of emotions. These include anxiety about uncertainties, doubt regarding negotiation outcomes, pessimism about diverse risks and negative scenarios, as well as concerns about the objectives, intentions, and trustworthiness of the other party.

The role of emotional intelligence has come to the fore in recent years due to the increasing turbulence of the environment. Recent economic instability and uncertainty have drastically affected people's emotional well-being, intensifying anxiety. All of this has given rise to profound concern about the future, as well as a feeling of insecurity regarding personal safety, social welfare, employment, and economic stability. The advance of digital technologies also has a dramatic impact on emotional stability, transforming the model for human interaction, especially for the younger generation. Technology is actually influencing the quality of interaction between people as well as their ability to empathize and understand other people's emotions.

As a result, the combination of these factors compels us to keep emotional intelligence in sharp focus when discussing business, teamwork, leadership, and of course, negotiation. For instance, research indicates that a leader with well-developed emotional intelligence not only enhances overall employee job satisfaction but also cultivates a positive work environment and fosters productivity and performance.

Emotional intelligence (or EI) can be defined in many ways. Most commonly, it refers to the ability to recognize and interpret one's own feelings, analyze emotional dynamics, and effectively manage and understand both personal emotions and those of others. The concept of EI has been extensively explored in psychological and organizational research due to its profound impact on personal and professional success. Today the role of EI is attracting more and more attention from researchers and practitioners. Daniel Goleman, a leading scholar in this field, divides emotional intelligence into five core components: 1) the capacity to identify and understand one's own emotions; 2) the ability to effectively manage and control one's emotional state and responses; 3) the capacity to channel emotions towards achieving personal goals; 4) the skill of recognizing and understanding the emotions of others; and 5) proficiency in managing interpersonal relationships and navigating the emotional dynamics of others.

Emotional intelligence is a non-cognitive skill which is increasingly considered one of the most essential for the future. In fact, according to the World Economic Forum's Future of Jobs Report 2025, characteristics originating from EI are among the most in-demand job skills moving forward. Indeed, an article that appeared in *Forbes* named emotional intelligence as number one skill for 2024.

There are several key components that lie at the heart of emotional intelligence. The first is *self-awareness*, which is the ability to understand our own emotions and how they influence our decisions and reactions. (In the case of negotiations, it can be helpful to identify what is an emotional trigger for you.) The second component is *self-regulation*, referring to the ability to control our emotions. *Social awareness* and *empathy* allow us to understand other people's emotions and how they affect their decisions and reactions.

Emotions often lead to unpredictable situations and have a profound impact on negotiations. It is worth recognizing that emotions can significantly change the outcome of negotiations. For example, research shows that the inability to adequately manage one's own emotions and the emotions of the other party leads to failure in negotiations.

Uncontrolled emotions can have dual consequences. On one hand, they may send unintended signals or offend the other party, damaging trust and long-term relations. On the other hand, they can cloud the negotiator's own judgment, hindering the ability to assess situations, respond appropriately, and make logical decisions. Mastering the art of emotional control is, therefore, an essential skill for effective negotiation. In this vein, when properly managed, emotions can become a powerful tool for communicating effectively, building trust, and achieving beneficial results.

Emotional control does not mean the absence of emotions but rather the tactical management of emotions. Yet some take the approach of simply ignoring emotions, as acknowledging them seems unprofessional. In practice, such an attitude is rarely fruitful and leads to unsuccessful negotiations. Imagine negotiators who are entirely devoid of emotion: for the other party, this would likely create a negative impression as they would appear cold, unapproachable, or even deceptive. As a result, such a lack of emotion could foster mistrust or frustration, damaging the negotiation process. For instance, if the situation calls for drawing attention to a particular issue, a negotiator might signal dissatisfaction with the direction of the discussion, or with a specific decision being taken. Emotions can be conveyed in various ways, such as through facial expressions, gestures, and other movements. It's crucial to be mindful of these signals, as the two parties will be observing one another's every move.

This discussion begs the question: "How can we successfully manage emotions?" There are diverse techniques to navigate emotional dynamics during a negotiation.

Let's start by first talking about a common emotion for negotiators: *anxiety*. Research indicates that anxiety is the dominant emotion during negotiations. Experiments demonstrate that anxiety may lead to the negotiator making less favorable offers, leaving the table sooner, reducing the speed of responses, agreeing to much less lucrative deals. Also, under the pressure of anxiety, a negotiator is more inclined to pass the decision on to other people. Other signs may also emerge too, such as halting speech or erroneous statements. We should keep in mind, however, that it's sometimes the negotiator's intent to induce a sense of unease in the other party.

So, how can we overcome anxiety? The first technique is to practice, turning negotiations into a habitual, everyday process. Anxiety often originates from the fact that negotiation is something new that rarely happens. Generally, novelty is a major source of anxiety, whether it's facing tests, assessments, or job interviews. When a situation shifts from unfamiliar and unique to familiar and routine, anxiety tends to diminish. In this regard, courses and negotiation training are a good solution for coping with anxiety, especially when they include practice sessions and negotiation simulations. Such training can dial down anxiety levels decisively, making individuals feel more confident and prepared.

Recognizing the reality of anxiety can also be helpful, as it's natural to feel uneasy when negotiation outcomes are uncertain. Thorough preparation helps to assuage anxiety too. When you've gathered and analyzed relevant information and developed a strategy and a clear plan, anxiety tends to lessen. Another effective technique is to focus on the negotiation process itself, setting aside concerns about the outcome temporarily. This shift in focus can alleviate the pressure that contributes to anxiety. Bringing a third party to the table can also be useful.

Anger can serve as both a natural response to an unsatisfactory proposal or offer in a negotiation, and as a tactical tool. Many negotiators perceive anger as a manifestation of power, a means to demonstrate dominance, and a method for putting on the pressure. Indeed, some negotiators still believe that there are positive sides of anger as a pressure tool which allows you to win a negotiation in the short-term. This emotion is especially prevalent in competitive strategy, where collaboration isn't a goal, nor is there any interest in fostering cooperation.

Anger has many negative effects on the negotiation process. It reduces the accuracy of proposals and impairs rationality. What's more, anger is not conducive to establishing long-term relations; it may also harm prospective future cooperation and leaves unpleasant feelings towards the negotiator who showed anger toward the other party. Overall, anger tends to erode trust between the negotiating parties.

Several techniques for dealing with anger are recommended. For example, when you're feeling angry, it's a good idea to take a break and give yourself time to calm down. The importance of stepping away momentarily should not be underestimated: this can be essential to recover your balance and manage your emotions. It's also helpful to refocus on the facts, as anger often leads to poor decisions and can distort your perception of the situation. When you're angry, try to control your tone too, because aggressive language can destroy trust. In general, if your goal is to create a collaboration and build a long-term partnership, then clearly you need to avoid anger or at least deal with it.

Although *joy* seems to be a positive emotion, it can also lead to negative consequences. For example, imagine the negotiation concluded very successfully for you – you secured all the advantages you were looking for and achieved all your objectives. Meanwhile, the other party, having made substantial concessions, fell short of their own goals. In this situation, openly demonstrating joy would only accentuate the other party's loss, amplifying their disappointment and dissatisfaction. Instead, it's wiser to exercise restraint and keep your emotions in check. Much like with anger, it's critical to stay focused on the facts to avoid becoming prematurely overjoyed, as this can negatively impact negotiation outcomes. However, joy can be tactically used to build trust, transforming warmth into genuine friendliness.

Disappointment can be both an unconscious expression of frustration with the negotiation process or its outcomes, and a conscious demonstration to encourage the other side to look at their behavior differently. It's advisable to remain objective in such situations. Is disappointment truly warranted or could the assessment be inaccurate? At times, disappointment can signal unfavorable negotiations, indicating it might be wise to change strategy.

Of course, in negotiations there are many other emotions that can have a pronounced impact on our behavior and on the other party, distorting our perceptions and consequently altering the results of negotiations.

Consequently, here are a few general recommendations for managing emotions.

TIPS FOR MANAGING EMOTIONS DURING NEGOTIATIONS

- Understand yourself; gain insight into your emotions, reactions, and behaviors in specific situations. Reflect on what triggers your responses and why you react the way you do.
- Understand others; cultivate empathy by trying to see the world from another person's perspective. Put yourself in their shoes to better comprehend their emotions and motivations.
- Take time to observe; allow yourself the time to listen attentively, notice subtle cues, and analyze situations thoughtfully. Avoid rushing to conclusions or decisions.

- Respect individuality; avoid projecting your own reactions, thoughts, or behaviors onto others. Recognize that each person perceives and responds to situations differently.
- Find out the root cause of negative emotions you may be sensing and try asking open-ended, general questions, such as "How is your day going?" "How will you get back home today?" "How's the weather where you live?"
- Don't take behaviors personally; understand that negative emotions are not directed at you as an individual but are a response to the situation or a reflection of the personal qualities of the other party involved in the negotiation.
- Avoid retaliating or trying to win; psychologists advise against escalating conflicts by responding to anger with anger.
- Reframe their words into neutral language; when the other party expresses themselves in a harsh or undiplomatic manner, translate their statements into a more neutral, inoffensive tone and respond accordingly.
- Create specific, measurable goals; focus on the content and try to engage the other party in it, distracting them from their emotions.

In general, it's also a good idea to ask yourself a few questions before starting a negotiation. Here are some examples: How am I feeling today? Should I express my emotions? What about the other party's feelings? What might happen in the negotiation that would make me angry? What might happen that would upset the other party? And finally, what do I expect from the negotiation, what results do I anticipate? How will I react to these results?

It's essential to realize that negotiation is a combination of the rational and emotional dimensions.

In the next chapter, we'll walk you through the role of communication in negotiation.

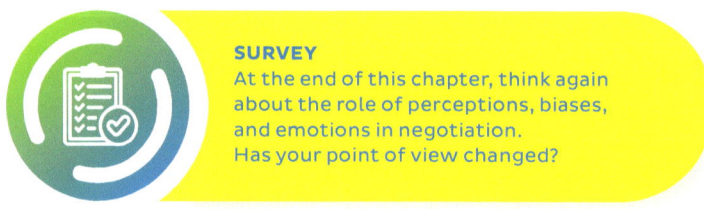

SURVEY
At the end of this chapter, think again about the role of perceptions, biases, and emotions in negotiation.
Has your point of view changed?

CHAPTER 4 | PERCEPTIONS, BIASES, AND EMOTIONS

VIDEO INTERVIEWS
Let's hear the experts' perspective on what influences perceptions and biases, how you can overcome them, and how to deal with the other party's emotions and your own while negotiating.

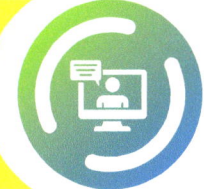

DIARY
Please take a moment to fill in your personal diary with your key takeaways.

READINGS
Here's a list of resources to help you learn more about this chapter's topics.

SUMMARY

BIASES

BIAS	DEFINITION	IMPACT ON NEGOTIATION	MANAGERIAL SUGGESTIONS
Confirmation bias	Focusing on information that confirms initial assumptions, ignoring data that support another point of view	The negotiator doesn't move forward; misses new opportunities.	• Analyze the whole stream of incoming information. • Consider what the other person is saying.
Anchor bias	Relying on the first piece of information you receive, allowing it to shape your judgment regardless of subsequent facts	The final decision is highly dependent on initial information; the negotiator loses objectivity.	• Gather and analyze all information. • Promote critical Thinking. • Set clear criteria.
Loss aversion	Avoiding losses at all costs	In trying to avoid any loss, the negotiator may miss more salient aspects of the negotiation.	• Don't overestimate losses. • Conduct a rational analysis of the negotiation and highlight the real value of the loss. • Outline a plan for what you can and cannot concede.

69

Overconfidence	A false sense of control, an illusion of optimistic outcomes	Overestimating your own position, which leads to ignoring risks, becoming less flexible, and possibly missing out on mutually beneficial opportunities.	• Engage outside opinions for objectivity. • Conduct thorough analyses of alternatives. • Acknowledge the likelihood of mistakes. • Prepare contingency plans.
Status quo	Perceiving a person with more authority or higher status as more influential, carrying more weight	Leads to losing objectivity; giving control in negotiations to the person who is higher in status.	• Focus on the facts. • Remain objective.

EMOTIONS

EMOTION	DEFINITION	IMPACT ON NEGOTIATION	MANAGERIAL SUGGESTIONS
Anxiety	Negative emotion of excitement, insecurity, uncertainty	Leads to making less favorable offers, leaving the negotiation sooner, reducing the speed of relevant reactions	• Recognize the reality of anxiety. • Be prepared for the negotiation. • Practice often and transform negotiations into a routine process. • Focus on the process, not on the outcome.
Anger	A negatively colored emotion and reaction expressed in resentment accompanied by facial expressions, body language	Possibly losing control, being less focused, missing important things Destroying long-term relationships, trust	• Take a break. • Focus on the facts. • Control your tone of voice.
Joy	Very positive emotion, feeling of fulfillment, pleasure and happiness	Can damage trust and long-term relationships	• Control the joy. • Stay focused. • Use joy to build trust.
Disappointment	Negative emotion, when reality doesn't meet hopes and expectations	Can derail decision-making and spoil the atmosphere of a negotiation	• Re-strategize. • Don't lose your objectivity.

EMOTIONAL CONTROL

EMOTIONAL CONTROL	MANAGERIAL SUGGESTIONS
Understand yourself.	Gain insight into your emotions, reactions, and behaviors in specific situations. Reflect on what triggers your responses and why you react the way you do.
Understand others.	Cultivate empathy by striving to see the world from another person's perspective. Put yourself in their shoes to better comprehend their emotions and motivations.
Take time.	Take time to observe and reflect, listen attentively, notice subtle cues, and analyze situations thoughtfully. Avoid rushing to conclusions or decisions.
Respect individuality.	Avoid projecting your own reactions, thoughts, or behaviors onto others. Recognize that each person perceives and responds to situations differently.
Find out the cause of the negative emotions.	Try asking open-ended questions, such as "How is your day going?" "How will you get back home today?" "How's the weather?"
Don't take behavior personally.	Understand that negative emotions are not directed at you as an individual but are a response to the situation or a reflection of the personal qualities of the other party involved in the negotiation.
Avoid retaliating or trying to win.	Psychologists advise against escalating conflicts by responding to anger with anger. For individuals who attempt to dominate through displays of anger, it is crucial to defuse their dominance without challenging their ego.
Reframe their words neutral language.	When the other party expresses themselves in a harsh or undiplomatic manner, translate their statements into a more neutral, inoffensive tone and respond accordingly.
Create specific, measurable goals.	Focus on the content and try to engage the other party in it, distracting them from their emotions.
Ask yourself a few questions.	Prepare for the main event, e.g., what might happen in the negotiation that would make me angry, what might happen that would upset the other party. And finally, think about: what I expect from the negotiation, what results I want to see, how I'll react to these results, whether I should express these feelings.

"Brevity is the soul of wit."
—WILLIAM SHAKESPEARE

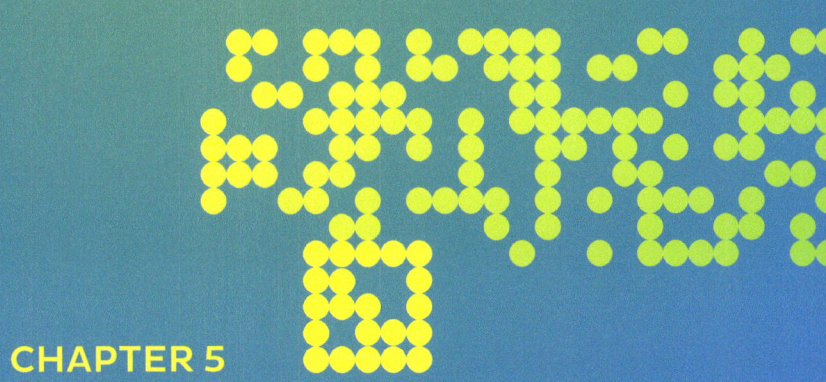

CHAPTER 5

COMMUNICATING EFFECTIVELY

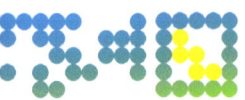

HOW IT WORKS

This chapter explores the main aspects of communication, both verbal and non-verbal, in the context of negotiation. We'll talk about the most common errors and how to overcome them. You'll be doing a series of online and off-line activities, such as reading, answering survey questions, watching video interviews, and writing in your diary. Below, you'll find detailed instructions on how to engage with this chapter of the book.

SURVEY
To start this chapter, this activity will get you thinking about communication errors that can come up in negotiations.

5.1 NON-VERBAL COMMUNICATION
In this section we'll analyze how non-verbal communication influences the overall dynamics of a negotiation.

5.2 VERBAL COMMUNICATION
Here we'll discuss the role of language and the art of asking questions, delving into the main types of questions.

5.3 COMMUNICATION ERRORS
In this section, you'll learn about typical communication errors, and get tips on how to overcome them when you're negotiating.

CHAPTER 5 | COMMUNICATING EFFECTIVELY

5.4 SHORT CASES

Here we present some short cases that illustrate the different communication traps discussed in the previous sections, along with recommendations for effectively dealing with them.

SURVEY
After reading this chapter, you may wish to reflect further on the most common communication errors in negotiations.

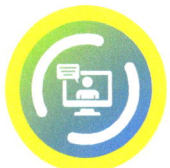

VIDEO INTERVIEWS
At this point you can watch the video interviews to hear the perspectives of experts on how to communicate effectively in negotiations.

DIARY
Please take a moment to fill in your personal diary with your key takeaways.

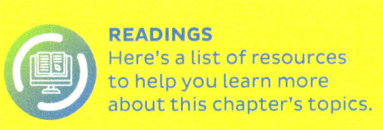

READINGS
Here's a list of resources to help you learn more about this chapter's topics.

SUMMARY

75

SURVEY
What are some communication errors that can come up during negotiations? Look at the list provided here and decide whether the items are serious communication errors in the context of negotiation.

5.1 NON-VERBAL COMMUNICATION

Communication is the tool through which any negotiation occurs. It is how intentions are expressed, proposals are made, and agreements are reached. Communication happens through non-verbal and verbal means, so only effective management of both dimensions can lead to successful negotiation dynamics and outcomes.

Non-verbal communication refers to modes of interaction that do not involve words. This serves as a powerful form of negotiation – sometimes even more impactful than speech. When you step into a negotiation room (whether or not it's a physical space), non-verbal communication speaks before you do. Your posture, gestures, and expressions reveal your intentions, reactions, and attitude, setting the tone and atmosphere for the entire process.

This form of communication has also played an incisive role throughout history. Napoleon, for example, is famous as a politician who actively used non-verbal communication. In the 19th century, during negotiations with Russian Emperor Alexander I and Prussian King Friedrich Wilhelm III, Napoleon shook his head at a key moment and signaled his complete disagreement with the proposal, showing his power, influence, and commanding position in the negotiations. The use of non-verbal communication is also prominently noted in the history of the 20th century. For example, during the negotiations between U.S. President John F. Kennedy and Soviet General Secretary Nikita Khrushchev at the UN Assembly in 1960, Khrushchev took off his shoe and banged it on the table. This gesture was a form of protest intended to demonstrate his dominance in the negotiations, signaling his dissatisfaction. Khrushchev's body language is famously recognized as a manifestation of his effort to take control over the political narrative.

Non-verbal communication includes things such as body language, proxemics and body contact, mirroring, clothing and appearance. The location of the negotiation is closely connected with non-verbal communication as well, as we'll see in the next section. Before we continue, we need to consider the role of perceptions and biases (discussed in detail in Chapter 4). In fact, what we need to keep in mind is that the signals conveyed through non-verbal communication may be interpreted differently by others and may not always align with the intent behind them.

Body language, one of the primary modes of non-verbal communication, includes posture, gestures, facial expressions, and eye contact.

Let's start with *posture*. An open posture demonstrates transparency and trust, creating a sense of receptivity. Leaning forward signifies interest, involvement, and positive emotion, showing engagement with the negotiation. Conversely, leaning back often conveys superiority, disdain, or perhaps disagreement.

Gestures can also deliver powerful messages. For instance, open palms reflect trust; on the contrary, crossed arms communicate closed mindedness, disagreement, domination. A hand on the heart indicates emotional involvement. In any case, as a general rule, the recommendation is to avoid excessive gesticulation, as it may create an impression of confusion or aggressiveness, which can be perceived as a lack of proper etiquette. Additionally, hand gestures can convey meaningful messages in the context of culture. (See Chapter 6 on culture in negotiations.) For instance, the "ok" gesture (thumbs up) in Western cultures means "everything is fine," but in South America it's a negative reaction to something. Putting your hands in your pockets may be an acceptable gesture in Western cultures, but in Japan it's an expression of disrespect and unprofessional behavior.

Not everyone is aware of how their *facial expressions* change, but controlling this aspect of non-verbal communication is vital. Facial expressions convey emotion, for instance, a smile indicates friendliness, a positive reaction to what you're hearing. An expression of surprise can reflect the fact that the information being discussed is unexpected for the other party, sometimes even unsatisfactory. An open facial expression helps create a friendly, comfortable atmosphere; conversely, a furrowed brow can generate tension. Be careful with indifferent facial expressions too, since that can be perceived as lack of interest in the negotiation and potentially in future cooperation.

Eye contact plays a salient role in building communication during a negotiation, but the meaning behind it depends a great deal on the cultural aspect of the context. In European culture, eye contact means openness, interest, and understanding. In Eastern cultures, instead, looking directly into someone's eyes can signal aggressiveness.

Attitudes about physical proximity and body contact can be conditioned both by the personal qualities of the negotiator (e.g., introvert/extrovert) and the cultural context. For example, during a negotiation, if you approach the negotiator representing the other party at a distance of 50 cm and engage in conversation in such close proximity, this can be considered inappropriate by an introvert or in certain cultural traditions. (For example, in Scandinavian countries people prefer to maintain more distance from others.)

Physical contact in some contexts may be a way to establish a warm atmosphere and friendly relations, while in others it may be considered a violation of traditions, etiquette, and personal space. What's more, in some cultures, touching is simply unacceptable or forbidden. So, when considering the appropriateness of physical contact (e.g., a handshake or touch on the shoulder), we must take into account both the personal preferences of the negotiator and the accepted business etiquette and cultural peculiarities. Therefore, proximity and physical contact must be carefully managed to avoid making the other party uncomfortable and giving rise to awkward situations.

Your clothing and appearance speak volumes about who you are and can send a powerful message. For example, if you dress informally for an important meeting, this can be seen as a lack of respect. Or showy, bright colored clothing can be perceived as a signal of dominance or disregard for accepted norms. For example, in the United States it's acceptable to come to a work event wearing a sweatshirt, but in Russia it would look disrespectful and unprofessional.

Mirroring the gestures and posture of the other party in a negotiation is a way to create a sense of rapport and establish a connection, putting everyone on the same wavelength. For example, if the other side is leaning forward, you can mimic this pose, showing that you are in the same emotional state and equally engaged in the negotiation process.

There are numerous recommendations regarding body language, some even suggesting serious training such as acting classes. Regardless of the approach, it's crucial to control your own body language while also observing that of the other party during negotiations. Assess and monitor your non-verbal communication. Consider making a video recording of yourself as you communicate. Then review and analyze your posture, gestures, facial expressions, and other non-verbal cues with the help of an expert.

Learn to pick up on the non-verbal signals of the other party during negotiations, too. Pay attention to signs of disagreement, satisfaction, interest, and other emotional responses. If you are sensing unfavorable non-verbal signals, it's worth delving into the root cause and possibly adjusting your style and strategy. Don't overload the negotiations with gestures and non-verbal signals, as this can be confusing and tiring for the other party. Manage your non-verbal communication and try to use it as a means to deliver signals and messages.

Active listening is a fundamental part of building an atmosphere of trust. If the other party perceives that they are not being listened to, or at least not attentively, this will diminish or even cancel out the effectiveness of the negotiation. (See Case 4 below about the power of active listening.) To demonstrate active listening, nod your head and use appropriate facial expressions to show your engagement and interest.

Be sensitive to cultural diversity. Above we've looked at some examples of how different cultures perceive non-verbal modes of communication differently. Pay attention and be well prepared if you have a cross-cultural meeting; specifically, learn what gestures, postures, facial expressions, and other non-verbal cues mean in various cultures.

5.1.1 Where to negotiate

The location of a negotiation can be considered a key part of non-verbal communication, as it greatly impacts the communication dynamic thanks to "a home field advantage," as the saying goes. Many politicians prefer to hold important meetings in their own country for this reason. In football, the outcome of a match can be influenced by whether the team is playing at home, with all the support of local fans, or away. For example, in the 1998 FIFA World Cup, the French football team won on their home turf thanks to this major psychological advantage. Similarly, in negotiation, a familiar environment reduces the levels of anxiety and stress. (See Chapter 4 about emotions.) Holding negotiations in your home territory also offers the advantage of support (if needed) from your colleagues, and allows you to control various aspects of the setting, such as seating arrangements and the choice of the meeting room. You can even organize lunch and coffee-breaks to create a more casual, relaxed atmosphere.

Moreover, inviting the other party to your home base can be a sign of hospitality, giving them the chance to experience your context and culture, e.g. organizing a company visit, proposing a city tour and a cultural program (e.g. museums and sightseeing). This approach can be an excellent way to establish positive relations and demonstrate goodwill.

By the same token, negotiation at your headquarters can also generate some risks for the other party. In fact, it could be used to employ pressure tactics, such as bringing in new stakeholders (the local press, experts, or public representatives), which can influence the dynamics of the negotiation.

Conversely, meeting the other party at their chosen venue for a negotiation may mean you'll be working in an unfamiliar environment. For instance, in these circumstances, you'd have little say over how the room is arranged, where everyone sits, or how the discussions are organized. You may also get tired from travelling back and forth from your home location. On the other hand, there are some advantages of negotiating in the home territory of the other party. For instance, agreeing to this shows your respect and willingness to collaborate; it gives you a change of scenery and distracts you from the daily routine of work and home, allowing you to concentrate fully on the discussion at hand. When travelling to another country for a negotiation, reading up on the cultural traditions is essential. (See Chapter 6 on the cultural dimension.)

Neutral territory for negotiations is often a good choice. This puts both parties on the same footing and can also help create a fairer, more balanced environment. Many historical political negotiations have been held in neutral territory. From the ancient world, we can look to the negotiations between Rome and Carthage (241 BC), which mostly took place in Sicily. In modern history, we can find examples too. For instance, in 1985 negotiations between the USSR and the US to end the Cold War were held in Geneva, Switzerland; the negotiation between Israel and Egypt in 1978 took place on American soil at Camp David.

5.2 VERBAL COMMUNICATION

Verbal communication includes all modes of interaction that use language, both spoken and written. Among the former, word choice, tone and questioning hold particular importance.

Regarding the use of spoken language, on the one hand, avoiding simplification is a must, while on the other, refraining from jargon and complex terms, obscure metaphors, or expressions unfamiliar to the other side is equally important. In a negotiation setting, you must clearly understand and articulate the message you wish to convey. Too often, instead of stating our message unambiguously, we resort to indirect communication such as jokes, innuendo, or leading questions, which can obscure our intentions, seriously risking creating misunderstandings.

Also powerful is the emotional coloring of your speech. (See Chapter 4 about emotions and emotional intelligence.) The same phrase expressed with different emotional undertones can be perceived differently. For example, communicating unpleasant news to the other party with empathy will help them accept it more calmly while feeling supported. If during negotiation you propose unfavorable conditions with indifference or with a smile, this could signal insensitivity to the other negotiators, and damage both your relationship with them and the negotiation process as a whole.

Language plays an especially critical role in multicultural and international communications (see Chapter 6). For example, "We can try this" in the US expresses openness to innovative approach, a willingness to try new things; but in Germany it conveys a lack of preparation and even disrespect. "It will be difficult" in England means that despite the challenge you are willing to work on it; in India the same expression reflects a negative attitude, telling the other party that you reject the idea. This being said, we have to remember that many things related to culture can be partly stereotypes. (Read more about this in Chapter 6.)

The course of the negotiation also largely depends on the art of questioning. There are several types of questions you can use when negotiating. Let's review the traditional classification.

Open-ended questions are valuable tools in negotiations, as they allow you to gather information, opinions, feelings, and perceptions from the other side. Usually these questions start with "what" or "how." But be aware that the responses may sometimes lack clarity or specificity, so it advisable to be prepared to follow up with other questions for a deeper dive into the topic. For example: "What do you think about the preliminary discussion we had last time?" or "Referring specifically to the level of quality, what would you consider excellent?"

It's best to phrase open-ended questions in a way that allows you to get maximum information. That's why you should avoid overly broad questions (e.g., "How is your firm doing?") and instead ask more specific ones (e.g., "What changes do you expect to see in your supply chain next January?").

There are some subtypes of open-ended questions, such as hypothetical, factual, opinion, and interest questions.

Hypothetical questions are useful for testing propositions, but they must remain grounded in reality. If such a question is based on unrealistic scenarios, it becomes ineffective and unhelpful. Here's an example of a hypothetical question: "If we were to offer you some additional services, how would this affect your decision?"

Factual questions and opinion questions can be useful as well. The choice between them depends on the context and your goals. Factual questions are crucial for clarifying terms, such as "What is the price of the product?"

Opinion questions serve to shape attitudes, build trust, and demonstrate that you care what the other party thinks. ("What do you think if we continue discussing discounts?")

Interest elicitation questions allow you to understand the real needs and interests of the other party, which can lead to long-term agreements. For instance, "What is important to you in this project?" Such questions help obtain more information, identify the underlying motivations behind decisions, and work together to find alternative solutions.

Closed questions let you get an unambiguous answer, save time, avoid assumptions, and minimize misunderstandings. On the other hand, the other side can feel cornered, as if you're giving them some sort of ultimatum. (For example: "Would you sign the agreement right now?") You should exercise caution when formulating closed questions, to ensure they don't sound intimidating, pressuring, or manipulating. Clarity is also key. Ensure your questions are specific. ("Do you agree with a price reduction of 10%?" rather than "Do you agree with this situation?")

Persistent questions can be useful to get more information, clarify arguments, and prompt a decision. At the same time, they may cause negative emotions in the other party and can be perceived as manipulation. Example: "What's the decisive factor for you when making your final decision?" This is how we would encourage the other side to show their hand and say what they need to conclude the deal.

Although direct questions are recommended since they leave no room for ambiguity and require concrete answers, such questions can create a negative impression on the other party, depending on their culture. (See Chapter 6.) Example: "What's your lowest price for this product?"

Multi-part questions combine several questions into one, making it possible to save time and achieve constructive progress more efficiently. However, they can sometimes create tension, intimidate, or confuse the other party. Often such questions are intended to identify additional opportunities to develop the deal and come to an agreement. Example: "If we could offer you a better price and provide supplementary products, how would that affect your decision to conclude this deal with us?" We would recommend using such questions with special care. If you put several questions into one, make sure to avoid information overload. This type of question is more appropriate when you need to get an answer on several factors: "What's more important to you, price, delivery time, or extra care?"

Particular attention should be given to written communication, since the written word is difficult to contest or retract. What's more, a written offer in some cases can equate to legal obligations. For example, if you're a concert organizer and you write to a celebrity to find out if they're free on a certain date, in some countries this simple written request means that you are obliged to invite the celebrity on that date.

Beyond this, you should formulate your thoughts clearly, avoiding errors and leaving no room for unintended interpretations that can lead to negative consequences. Example: "We will complete the repair work in three months, but deadlines may vary depending on circumstances." This is too vague; it doesn't specify *which* circumstances or *how* exactly the deadlines may change. Such a statement can lead to disputes and even legal action. As for the positive side of written communication, you have time to think about your answers, analyze the situation, and come up with alternatives, whereas in oral communication there is often little or no time to do all this.

5.3 COMMUNICATION ERRORS

Below, we'll look at some typical communication errors made during negotiations and tips on how to overcome them.

Very often *insufficient preparation* for negotiations leads to serious mistakes. The importance of preliminary work to determine how to communicate effectively cannot be overestimated. Gathering information about the other party's communication approach and analyzing your own strengths and weaknesses is fundamental to successful negotiations.

A common mistake is *failing to pay proper attention to non-verbal communication*. As with other aspects of negotiation, preparation is key when it comes to non-verbal communication as well. It's crucial to analyze your own non-verbal cues, including your facial expressions and appearance, while also closely observing the non-verbal signals from the other party.

Verbal communication is obviously the heart of communication in negotiation. *Failing to approach verbal communication with the necessary seriousness* is a mistake many negotiators make. In verbal communication, clarity is essential; sentences should be logical and easy to understand, avoiding any ambiguity. As we've said before, negotiations are a dialogue, not a monologue. Talking excessively and dominating the conversation while the other party merely listens is not the best approach. Effective negotiations thrive on a balanced discussion between both parties. If you monopolize the conversation all the time, you won't be able to understand what the other party is looking for, and you can also make a very negative impression. Also avoid interrupting, as it can be extremely frustrating for the other party. Lastly, it is vital to formalize agreements to ensure that there is mutual understanding and accountability.

A major mistake in negotiations is *underestimating the importance of active listening.* Other than establishing a positive relationship, actively listening to the other party also allows you to gather valuable information; it fosters a positive atmosphere and encourages the dialogue to move forward. Combined with the ability to carefully process information, active listening offers critical advantages and supports the overall negotiation process. This skill also conveys respect, engagement, and genuine interest. To show you are actively listening to the other party, you can take notes, summarizing key points after each topic, and emulate their language and expressions. This kind of mirroring encompasses both verbal cues, such as affirming with phrases like "I see," or "That makes sense," and non-verbal cues, including nodding, maintaining eye contact, and adopting an open posture.

Very often we *focus on what to say next*, instead of carefully listening to and understanding the arguments of the other party. We sometimes worry about how to articulate our next point or ensure that we convey something pertinent. However, failing to truly understand what the other side is saying undermines effective communication. If you don't concentrate on the other party's points, but give your own pre-prepared speech, they may get a sense of disrespect, that you're not taking their arguments into account.

Don't try to *present everything all at once*. Information overload, giving too much irrelevant or overly detailed input, can lead to negative emotions, irritation, and stress for the other party. Even if it's important, it's worth remembering that the other party is not always able to remember or process large amounts of information.

Another major communication mistake is *not paying attention to emotional vibes*. This may happen if we're too concentrated on ourselves. In this vein, it's advisable to find a better balance between focusing inward and outward. As shown in Case 3 below, if you sense negative emotions on the other side, you should react accordingly. Also, when emotions are running high, taking a break can be a good solution. Emotions occupy a separate place in the communication process, and an inability to manage emotions can disrupt the entire negotiation. If you are a highly emotional negotiator, then it would be useful to be part of a team, not to fly solo. If roles are properly assigned, beginning as a team can help you mitigate and better manage your own emotions. It's also a must to keep a neutral tone, avoiding aggression or sarcasm. Try to use emotions as a resource, so if you show confidence and a positive attitude, it will create a positive atmosphere.

The *time for negotiations* must be carefully considered. We all aim to achieve results quickly. However, rushing through without taking the time to thoroughly discuss the terms and explore all the details of a potential deal is unwise. Such haste can result in costly mistakes.

Honesty is an essential part of building trust in communication. So *do not make promises that you can't keep*. In practice, we realize that false promises will sooner or later lead to a breakdown of relations, trust and reputation between negotiators and eventually organizations.

Conducting negotiations *without considering the cultural context* can represent a critical mistake. The cultural factor has considerable impact on communication (discussed in more detail in Chapter 6). Both kinds of communication, but especially non-verbal, may be perceived differently in different cultures. In addition, certain cultures may prioritize specific styles and nuances of negotiation. In multicultural negotiations, we recommend adapting to the communication style of the other party; pay attention to whether they prefer a direct or indirect communication style. In case of an international negotiation conducted in foreign language, it is advisable to avoid complex grammatical constructions. Try to speak clearly, using simple, direct language.

Today, a new form of communication has emerged: digital communication, or more precisely phygital communication. It is a critical error to *ignore the nuances of communication in the phygital world*, which we'll explore in Chapter 7.

Here, we'll simply say that negotiations in the phygital world have evolved, and it's crucial to consider the interplay between digital and non-digital elements in the process. Ensuring adequate technical support is necessary to avoid issues such as communication breakdowns during negotiations. In a phygital environment, professionalism is key, for instance, adhering to a dress code and minimizing background noise during video calls. Maintaining high standards of professionalism is equally essential both offline and online. It's also helpful to use digital tools even in offline negotiations, as a means of support and a quick channel for communication. Staying updated with technological advancements, utilizing contemporary tools and software, and continuously enhancing professional skills: these are keys to success in modern negotiations.

In the next chapter, we will look at how the multicultural and international dimensions affect the dynamics of negotiating.

5.4 SHORT CASES

CASE 1 OPEN-ENDED QUESTIONS

Two companies are engaged in negotiations regarding renting various properties. Company A wants to organize a festival and rent a big hall from Company B. Although, based on some market analysis, they have the leeway to offer up to €70 thousand, Company A begins the negotiation by proposing €50 thousand. Company B perceives this as disinterest in their own needs, and responds by adopting a distributive strategy, answering that the rent is €70 thousand, non-negotiable. As a result, the negotiations reach an impasse.

A key recommendation in this case would be to apply open-ended questions. Let's reset the scene. Company A follows this approach and starts asking questions, such as: "Why is it so important for you that the rent be set at €70 thousand? Do we have any other options?" The representative of Company B answers that they are somewhat worried about the safety of the hall. Company A then proposes to reduce the rent to €60 thousand, while also taking on the responsibility of securing an insurance contract for the hall that covers all risks. Company B accepted this offer, since in their view it would be an effective risk mitigation solution.

In the end, the negotiation results in a beneficial outcome for both parties. In shifting from a distributive strategy to an integrative one (as discussed in Chapter 3), both parties have found a joint creative solution that meets their primary goals and lays the foundations for future collaborations.

CASE 2 BODY LANGUAGE

Negotiations are taking place between the Marketing Department (headed by Peter) and the HR Department (headed by Simona). The subject is budget allocations. Initially, the negotiation is very tense, the atmosphere is uncomfortable and charged with negative emotions. Peter is sitting back, arms crossed, brow furrowed. He claims that Simona's department always gets more funding, which is unfair, and it's time to shift priorities in favor of his department. Simona also crosses her arms and shakes her head. She argues that from her perspective the situation is fair because her department is exposed to a high level of uncertainty and, consequently, as priorities suddenly change, they need to get more funds.

In this case, the most effectual recommendation is to change body language and facial expressions. Taking this into account, Peter sits with open palms, smiles, and maintains eye contact. He acknowledges to Simona that he understands she is pressed for time and asks if available funds can be allocated in a way that allows both departments to meet their goals. Simona says she's open to starting a constructive conversation about the budget allocation. In the end, they agree to have a conversation prior to any extra-budget request. This way they can size such a request according to the needs of both parties.

This case demonstrates that non-verbal communication, when used appropriately, can alleviate tension and facilitate communication. Conversely, a lack of positive non-verbal cues can create pressure and lead to an impasse in the negotiation process.

CASE 3 **THE POWER OF BREAKS**

Negotiations are underway to extend the employment contract with an expert in finance. The employee is requesting a 10% salary increase and change in position from Head of Finance to Deputy Finance Director. The HR Director insists that this is not possible. Several emotional declarations follow, along with negative non-verbal cues; the situation gets tense, and the negotiation reaches an impasse. The recommendation here is to take a break, to calm down and put the info together, review what's going on, what's missing, what to ask for more information, how to refocus the goal of the meeting. After the break, tempers have cooled, and both parties start asking several questions to better understand the reasoning of the other person. After gathering more information, they then decide to proceed with the negotiation applying an integrative strategy. So, the HR Director asks what the priority is and what can create additional value for the employee, who responds that for her, the new position is what counts most. As a result, they agree to the position of Deputy Finance Director, but with no pay raise.

In this case we see how a break allows negotiators to release tension, to analyze the situation, and to find a joint solution.

CASE 4 **ACTIVE LISTENING**

Company A is a large luxury clothing manufacturer planning to integrate artificial intelligence into its business processes. So Company A invites Company B, which is specialized in AI, to collaborate. The representative of Company A (Jorge) shares their plans and expectations for project implementation. The representative of Company B (Gary) is checking his phone as Jorge speaks. Jorge asks if Gary is listening. Gary responds, "Yes, go ahead, I can check my phone and listen at the same time." Jorge gets angry and stops talking; the negotiation reaches an impasse.

Recommendations here would be for Gary to put his phone away and use active listening (e.g., nodding, using phrases like "I see" or "Tell me more," taking notes) to demonstrate engagement, respect, and willingness to cooperate.

In the end, Gary follows this advice and listens actively. Jorge feels heard and respected. He also realizes that his request and his interests are being taken seriously. As a result, the negotiation becomes collaborative. The parties agree to initiate a joint project and work together to draft an agreement detailing the services Gary's company will provide to Jorge's company for the adoption of an AI system.

This case illustrates the pivotal role of active listening in building rapport and fostering productive negotiations. On the contrary, the absence of active listening can hinder the progress of negotiations and damage relations between the parties.

CASE 5 — INFORMATION OVERLOAD

Here we find Jack, the founder of a start-up, negotiating with Mark, a potential investor. Jack spends an hour discussing his company, covering a wide range of topics, including technical details, logistics, financing, and marketing strategies. Jack is sharing tons of information, and this is creating stress and anxiety for Mark. In these settings, we can recommend that Jack outline his request and interests in writing, for example, using a shared whiteboard and presenting some notes while the meeting is progressing, to help Mark get a better grasp of what's going on. Jack takes the recommendations into account, makes his request and interests more structured, reduces the number of minor details, and writes on a whiteboard to illustrate the complex technical issues impacting his start-up. As a result, Mark gains a clearer understanding of the company, reducing his confusion and stress. This clarity leads to an agreement on funding the start-up.

In the end, reducing information overload helps to diminish negative emotions, and foster collaborative negotiations and beneficial outcomes for all parties.

SURVEY
After reading this chapter, reflect on the most common communication errors in negotiations. See how your perspective has changed.

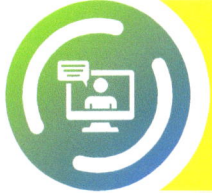

VIDEO INTERVIEWS
How much of communication is influenced by culture, age, working experience? We ask this and other questions to experts and learn their recommendations for communicating effectively.

DIARY
Please take a moment to fill in your personal diary with your key takeaways.

READINGS
Here's a list of resources to help you learn more about this chapter's topics.

SUMMARY

NON-VERBAL COMMUNICATION	Modes of interaction that do not involve words: • body language (eye contact, posture, gestures, and facial expressions) • proxemics and physical contact • appearance • mirroring • location
RECOMMENDATIONS ON NON-VERBAL COMMUNICATION	• Analyze and monitor your non-verbal communication. • Learn to observe the non-verbal signals of the other party. • Do not overload the negotiations with gestures and non-verbal signals. • Listen actively. • Be sensitive to cultural diversity.
VERBAL COMMUNICATION	All forms of interaction that use language, both spoken and written; for spoken verbal communication, word choice, tone, and questioning hold particular importance.

QUESTION TYPES	• Open-ended
	  - hypothetical
	  - factual
	  - opinion
	  - interest
	• Closed
	• Persistent
	• Direct
	• Multi-part

COMMUNICATION ERRORS	• Not preparing adequately • Failing to pay attention to non-verbal communication • Failing to properly consider verbal communication • Underestimating the importance of active listening • Focusing on what to say next, instead of carefully listening • Presenting everything at once • Not paying attention to emotional vibes • Rushing negotiations • Making promises that cannot be kept • Ignoring cultural context • Neglecting the nuances of communication in the phygital world

"No one is an island."
_JOHN DONNE

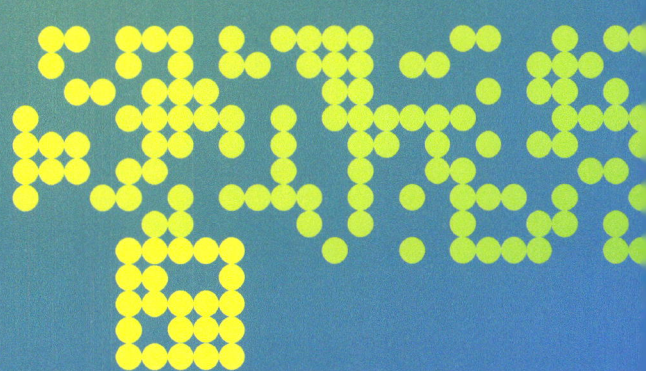

CHAPTER 6

MULTICULTURAL AND INTERNATIONAL SETTINGS

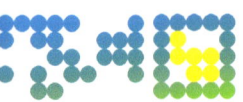

HOW IT WORKS

In today's increasingly globalized world, there are more opportunities – and a greater need – to develop partnerships with stakeholders from different countries and cultures than ever before. But along with exciting prospects come momentous challenges, particularly in the setting of multicultural and international negotiations. Navigating the differences that arise, one of the biggest obstacles, can critically influence the effectiveness of a negotiation. With this in mind, the chapter aims to explore how multicultural and international dimensions shape negotiation dynamics, outlining the main characteristics of negotiations with international institutions, and highlighting how critical it is to prepare for similar settings. To do all this, you'll have a series of activities, such as reading the static sections and working on dynamic activities online (survey questions, video interviews, and diary). Below, you'll find detailed instructions on how to engage with this chapter of the book.

SURVEY
To start out this chapter, you'll be invited to reflect on the most relevant dimensions that can influence multicultural and international negotiations.

6.1 FRAMING MULTICULTURAL AND INTERNATIONAL NEGOTIATIONS
We'll discuss the main differences between the two.

6.2 NEGOTIATIONS WITH INTERNATIONAL INSTITUTIONS
This section intends to increase your awareness of some peculiarities of international institutions.

6.3 STEREOTYPES SHAPE REALITY

We'll elaborate on the phenomenon of stereotypes, their origins, and their role in negotiations.

6.4 HOW TO PREPARE FOR MULTICULTURAL AND INTERNATIONAL NEGOTIATIONS

In this section, we'll present indispensable advice on how to properly prepare for multicultural and international negotiations.

SURVEY
At the end of the chapter, you'll be asked to reflect again on the dimensions that can influence negotiations in multicultural and international settings.

VIDEO INTERVIEWS
You can now watch the video interviews to hear experts offer their perspectives.

DIARY
Please take a moment to fill in your personal diary with your key takeaways.

READINGS
Here's a list of resources to help you learn more about this chapter's topics.

SUMMARY

SURVEY
Before continuing to read, think about the different dimensions that can influence the effectiveness of a multicultural and international negotiation and rate them based on their relevance.

6.1 FRAMING MULTICULTURAL AND INTERNATIONAL NEGOTIATIONS

The phenomena of globalization and rapid advances in technologies are bringing the world closer together. Nowadays, we can connect with someone on the other side of the world via videocall in a matter of seconds, send a package from Latin America to Europe in days, or purchase fruit from South Africa in a store in Finland.

When doing business in such international contexts, there are numerous elements to consider, such as environmental factors, foreign bureaucracies, divergent processes, laws, and financial constraints. One of the elements that can become a barrier is cultural contrasts. In fact, different cultures may interpret the same expressions, phrases, and gestures in different ways. Effective negotiators must ensure that culture does not become a divisive factor. Instead, it should serve as a bridge and help enrich collaborations.

In this context, the forces of globalization and cultural diversity are shaping our lives, communication dynamics, business relations, and the way we negotiate with one another. For instance, as far as conflict resolution, the Japanese culture tends to prioritize an indirect, cooperative style, whereas North Americans are more likely to solve conflict in a direct, win-lose style.

It's essential at this point to clarify what we mean by multiculturalism and internationality. Multiculturalism is the existence of many cultures, traditions, habits, and peculiarities. Basically, it is the backbone for collaboration with individuals from various cultural backgrounds. We face multiculturalism not only when negotiating with representatives from other countries, but also from the same country, as we work in multicultural teams and appreciate the richness of diverse cultures. Multiculturalism calls for preserving and respecting cultural identities, while learning from the diversity around us. Internationality refers to strengthening international cooperation and unity between different cultures and peoples. In part, the international dimension also encompasses multiculturalism.

While multicultural negotiations can be held in a single country, the composition of the negotiation team may be multinational. This means that international negotiations are not necessarily about different cultures, but the parties acting in different countries. In this vein, a conditional distinction is applied here, where multicultural dimensions (such as cultures, traditions, and languages differences) are addressed separately, while challenges related to time zones, technical issues, and technological constraints fall under the international dimensions of negotiation.

6.1.1 Multicultural negotiations

Given the diversity of cultures that exist on our planet, it's crucial to understand, appreciate, and respect the relevant differences. Cultural dimensions influence both multicultural and international negotiations, but in the former the effect is more keenly felt. So the question arises as to how we can truly understand and consider all cultural nuances. In response, several models for "measuring" national cultures have been developed, offering practical tools for analyzing cultural differences in various processes, including negotiations. By providing insights into key cultural dimensions, these models enable us to gain a deeper understanding of how to navigate and respect diverse cultural perspectives in a global environment.

According to Institutional Theory, the cultural-cognitive influence on individual and organizational behavior comprises our collective understanding of what social reality is, and provides the prism through which we interpret information. Culture, as the "collective programming of the mind" transmitted across generations, shapes the way individuals within a society think, feel, and behave.[1] By molding personal cognitions and informing the attribution of meaning and value to motivational factors, culture guides individuals' choices, commitments, and behaviors (including what happens in negotiations). This process affects how people perceive situations, make decisions, and interact with others, impacting negotiations across different cultural contexts.

As mentioned above, researchers propose several models to evaluate cultural dimensions. One of the most interesting in the context of negotiations is Global Leadership and Organizational Behavioral Effectiveness (GLOBE), which was created by Robert House in 1991.[2] This model identifies nine cultural dimensions that explain the differences in values, behaviors, and practices across various cultures. Below, we present how these dimensions may impact negotiations.

Uncertainty avoidance is defined as "the extent to which members of an organization or society strive to avoid uncertainty by reliance on social norms, rituals, and bureaucratic practices to alleviate the unpredictability of future events."[3] If in a negotiation this is a cultural trait of one of the parties, they will be less inclined to accept risky propositions or innovation. Furthermore, any uncertainties, or any chancy or even original proposals can drastically complicate negotiations. In risk-averse cultures, stability and peaceful negotiations, as well as harmonious relationships with partners, are often prioritized and secure, predictable outcomes are normally favored.

Power distance reflects "the degree to which members of an organization or society expect and agree that power should be unequally shared."[4] In cultures where power-distance is high, negotiators may have limited authority to make decisions and little freedom of action during negotiations, so they have to coordinate with their superiors. Also, such cultures tend not to accept innovations when they are inclined to respect a rigid hierarchy. In such cultures, the style of negotiation is more formal, official, and less personal.

Societal collectivism is "the degree to which organizational and societal institutional practices encourage and reward collective distribution of resources and collective action."[5] Obviously, with a high level of collectivism, negotiators from such cultures will probably be less autonomous in their decision-making, and more likely to think in terms of benefits for the organization rather than personal advantages. In these cultural contexts, access to resources is limited and controlled; shared group goals and objectives are the priority. Additionally, individual ideas are not highly valued; negotiators have less freedom, less creativity, and less orientation toward innovative behavior. On the contrary, in cultures with a low level of collectivism, there is more freedom, stronger orientation towards personal interests, and more individual authority and creativity.

In-group collectivism reflects "the degree to which individuals express pride, loyalty and cohesiveness in their organizations or families."[6] Cultures with low value of in-group collectivism tend to emphasize independent decision-making, with a strong desire for autonomy and freedom. In such cultures, it's often expected that individuals prioritize their personal interests and goals. So when negotiating with people from these cultures, it's beneficial to respect and engage the individual's unique perspective, crafting a personalized cultural program and employing specific techniques that resonate with that person's values.

Gender egalitarianism is "the extent to which an organization or a society minimizes gender role differences and gender discrimination."[7] We must be very attentive to gender in general. In some cultures, certain actions are simply driven by etiquette, while in other cultures the same actions may be perceived as offensive and discriminatory (e.g., handing someone your coat, letting people pass ahead of you).

Assertiveness is "the degree to which individuals in organizations or societies are forceful, confrontational, or aggressive in social relationships."[8] People from cultures where strong assertiveness is the norm are willing to take risks, engage in non-collaborative negotiation tactics, and foster competitive negotiation. In such contexts, the primary goal of negotiation is often more important than maintaining long-term relationships. In contrast, cultures with low assertiveness view negotiation as collaboration, emphasizing the need to consider the interests of all parties involved. Here, negotiations are seen as a peaceful, cooperative process aimed at finding win-win solutions and building long-term relations.

Future orientation is defined as "the degree to which individuals in organizations or societies engage in future-oriented behaviors such as planning, investing in the future, and delaying gratification."[9] Societies that value such an orientation focus on future success and enduring relationships. As we've previously discussed (Chapter 2), negotiations are often a choice, a balance between maximizing value in the short-term perspective and building a long-term relationship with a partner. It's obvious that in cultures with a high degree of future orientation, the priority is working toward strategic goals, long-term relationships and prospective plans.

Performance orientation is "the extent to which an organization or society encourages and rewards group members for performance improvement and excellence."[10] In a similar context, initiative, hard work, competitiveness, challenging goals, and results are valued. Accordingly, negotiators strive to achieve results. They are also more inclined to adopt a competitive or distributive negotiation strategy than a collaborative one. (See also Chapter 3.)

Humane orientation is the extent to which people in organizations or societies encourage and reward individuals for fairness, altruism, friendliness, generosity, caring and kindness to others.[11] In similar cultures, people access resources and necessary social support from their immediate environment and display a high degree of conformity. As a result, negotiators from this culture are more likely to compromise and prioritize good relationships.

What clearly emerges from the descriptions above is that properly addressing these cultural characteristics can significantly improve negotiation effectiveness.

6.1.2 International negotiations

As we pointed out above, cultural dimensions are salient factors in negotiations, both multicultural (to a greater extent) and international (to a lesser extent). Focusing on the international dimension, some specific elements emerge, such as language barriers, time zone differences, technology-related issues, and even gastronomic preferences. Let's take a closer look at each of these points.

Although it may seem obvious, *language barriers* should not be underestimated in negotiations. Different languages often convey varying degrees of enthusiasm and expressions of agreement, dissatisfaction or joy. These nuances in native languages can also be reflected when a negotiator is speaking in a foreign language. In fact, even a conversation in English can be perceived differently – more emotionally intense for some cultures, more reserved for others. In general, when negotiating in a non-native language, we often tend to mentally translate from our mother tongue, which can lead to carrying nuances of meaning and even emotional undertones that differ from the original intention. Additionally, when negotiations involve an interpreter, we must be particularly attentive. It's crucial to prepare the interpreter thoroughly beforehand, explaining the nature and context of the negotiations to ensure more accurate communication. Considering language differences is essential to accurately interpret the signals being sent by the other party during negotiations.

Diverse interpretations of emotions, movements, and behaviors can also create obstacles. For example, laughing in European cultures is generally a sign of pleasure, satisfaction, or happiness, while in Japanese culture, it often reflects nervousness, embarrassment, or an attempt to mask discomfort. Attitudes toward punctuality also vary greatly. In Italy, being 15 minutes late for lunch is socially acceptable, while in Scandinavian countries, it's considered disrespectful and rude.

Technical barriers can affect negotiations too, such as differences in time zones. Although this may seem like something simple, it can have a substantial impact on the negotiation process. We need to be mindful of such details when scheduling meetings, for instance, avoid setting times that may require the other party to join a call at 3:00 a.m. on their side of the world.

With online negotiations, *technological issues* can arise, for example, certain video conference systems may be inaccessible or even banned in some countries, creating barriers to communication. Being aware of these challenges and addressing them in advance can help get things started on the right foot and ensure more effective negotiations.

When negotiators come from different countries for an in-person meeting, *gastronomic considerations* can play an important role. It's crucial to avoid any serious mistakes, for example, serving food or beverages that are forbidden or considered inappropriate for some of the negotiators.

Finally, we need to pay attention to *etiquette*, which can vary greatly by country and culture. Etiquette includes norms and rules concerning different aspects of communication and life, norms of behavior in public places and in the workplace, forms of greeting and conversation, and appropriate dress. What's more, etiquette applies to both verbal and non-verbal communication. For instance, in many European cultures, maintaining eye contact with your interlocutor is customary, while in some Eastern cultures, it may be considered inappropriate. In China, punctuality often means arriving slightly earlier than the scheduled time, whereas in Scandinavian countries, arriving precisely at the agreed time is perfectly acceptable. In addition, standards of digital etiquette are currently emerging, and although several global norms exist today, in the digital space there are still a few peculiarities. For example, for some negotiators it's customary to get straight to the point in online negotiations, while it's not the case for others.

Ensuring that these details align with local customs is a way to demonstrate respect. Such efforts can help to develop solid relationships, as manners and conversation styles are often seen as reflections of negotiators' professionalism, friendliness, and cultural awareness.

6.2 NEGOTIATION WITH INTERNATIONAL INSTITUTIONS

A critical scenario may arise in multinational and international contexts when we need to negotiate with international institutions, such as governments, state or supranational organizations, or diplomatic agencies. Topics to address might be the terms of general policies, product quality requirements, compliance with legislative norms, a commercial memorandum of understanding, or even a peace treaty, just to mention a few.

For example, a Mexican company might negotiate with the Chinese Ministry of Commerce to reduce tariffs on agricultural exports; a European energy company may negotiate with a representative of the Indian government on terms for the construction of a solar power plant; a European pharmaceutical company can negotiate through its embassy with the Indonesian government to resolve a licensing dispute.

In general, international institutions do not perceive themselves as negotiating entities, as companies would in the business world. This is primarily because these bodies operate strictly within an established set of rules and, as official representatives of a central authority, they possess significant advantages and sources of power.

When negotiating with business organizations, usually we have more options, e.g., to walk away, or to switch to another company. However, when negotiating with a government, such choices are often limited. Governments do not rely heavily on the outcome of a single deal, as they are not dependent on the income generated from it. (Instead, their income comes from regular tax revenues.)

For international institutions, public interest plays a crucial role in any negotiation process. Moreover, these bodies operate under special procedures and regulations. They place great importance on preserving prestige and status, often doing so through formal protocols, behaviors, and transactional norms.

Considering these sources of negotiating power, how do we approach negotiations with international institutions and governments? Below you'll find recommendations based on the literature.

TIPS FOR APPROACHING NEGOTIATIONS WITH INTERNATIONAL INSTITUTIONS

- **Be prepared.** You must thoroughly understand the laws, regulations, rules and bureaucratic procedures of the institution you intend to negotiate with. For example, a large tech company might want to negotiate with the European Commission on the compliance of its technological services with GDPR requirements (General Data Protection Regulation). As we know, data security and privacy are top priority for the European Commission. Consequently, demonstrating a high level of preparedness and clear understanding of GDPR rules would be a key negotiation element for the tech company.

- **Demonstrate respect.** Showing respect for the status of the other party, as well as the applicable laws and the institution they represent, is essential. For example, let's say a company from the European Union intends to negotiate with the Singapore government to establish a venture focused on video gaming. During the negotiations, the EU company should show its respect for Singapore's long experience in technology development, specifically in the gaming industry.

- **Find a precedent.** Experienced negotiators recommend researching similar deals that have been done before. In other words, it's helpful to find comparable situations or requests from other companies where the institution has supported a similar decision. For example, let's take a Spanish company that's planning to develop a creative space in a former factory building; it's discussing this possibility with the municipal government of a city in Argentina. The company aims to establish a public-private partnership, but the government is hesitant. For the Spanish private company, profit is a primary objective, whereas the government prioritizes public service, sustainability, and long-term benefits. To persuade the government, the company conducts an analysis highlighting several successful cases of similar partnerships. These examples demonstrate how city authorities supported programs to repurpose factory buildings, transforming them into creative spaces that generated not only profits for private partners but also significant benefits for the city and its residents.

- **Showcase diverse impacts.** Demonstrating the broader impact of your proposal is also effective. Rather than presenting it solely as a commercial venture (such as opening a factory or shopping mall), it's essential to emphasize its social benefits. For instance, you could stress how the project will contribute to reducing crime or provide young people with engaging entertainment options, such as cafes or cinemas. For another example, in terms of social benefits, the Indonesian Health Department and a Spanish health company are negotiating on establishing a network of clinics in Indonesia. The Health Department is mostly concerned about the public reaction; transparency represents a key driver. Consequently, publicizing the initiative and explaining its high social impact would be well received by the public.

- **Focus on the human factor.** The importance of relationship-building cannot be overstated. When you negotiate with an international institution, it's useful to keep in mind that there are individuals in positions of authority; also remember that the human factor, along with emotions, both play a role in the process.

6.3 STEREOTYPES SHAPE REALITY

When discussing multicultural and international negotiations, it's impossible to overlook the role of stereotypes. In fact, stereotypes have been identified by a number of researchers as factors that significantly affect the management of multicultural and international communication processes, teams, and negotiations.

It's often hard to draw the line between reality and stereotypes, making it complicated to differentiate between the two. As a result, we frequently rely on stereotypes rather than truths. So what are stereotypes? Cultural and national stereotypes refer to a widely accepted belief: that people from the same place share a set of common features of behavior. Stereotyping is a cognitive process of categorization, which gives rise to general attitudes toward a certain group of people.

The source of the stereotyping mechanism originates from a primitive human instinct to separate the group into "one of us/not one of us," "dangerous/not dangerous." Researchers assert that when we stereotype, the main question we ask ourselves (subconsciously, of course) is whether the other person can or wants to do us harm. This mechanism, rooted in our ancient evolution, was essential for survival. Stereotyping made it simple to rely on basic traits rather than a deep analysis of a group of people. The need for quick decision-making meant that this approach was both efficient and necessary. Accordingly, stereotyping is primitivization, simplification, reduction of the whole cultural diversity to a rather simple set of behavioral traits of a certain group (to include traditions, habits, experience, history, literature, gastronomy, geography, and many other things that influence the formation of culture). Stereotypes about a group of people usually rely on certain simple, easily identifiable characteristics, such as age, nationality, or occupation (all professors, all young people, all Americans, and so on). It's interesting that even if stereotypes don't correspond to reality, they tend to be very stable, influential, and hard to overcome.

Stereotypes have something in common with fairy tales and myths, with similar mechanisms of simplification, hyperbolization, creation of clear roles and division of work. What's more, some stereotypes are shaped by masterpieces of the arts such as literature and cinema. Indeed, artistic creations often leave a lasting imprint on our perceptions of different countries. For example, the adventures of Sherlock Holmes by Arthur Conan Doyle have significantly influenced how people view the inhabitants of Great Britain, while Federico Fellini's films have played a key role in shaping the global perception of Italians. These artistic images contribute to forming and reinforcing national cultural stereotypes.

Stereotypes vary in intensity: some are not widely accepted, while others are deeply rooted in our shared perceptions. In some cases, stereotypes become so powerful that they hold more sway than objective facts. When individuals rely on stereotypes, the phenomenon of prejudice emerges. In addition, some stereotypes are shaped by perceived and actual economic, geographic, and normative factors, as well as power dynamics. These aspects can contribute to the formation of beliefs that may not reflect reality. Everything we've mentioned above is crucial to remember to approach negotiations with a more open and informed mindset.

6.3.1 Examples of stereotypes for multicultural and international negotiations

G. Richard Shell, in his book *Bargaining for Advantage* (2006), gives an example of a negotiation between British and Lebanese parties. The British negotiators offered several concessions and received worse terms on the proposed deal in return. So they refused to negotiate further, but then received several offers from the Lebanese side with much better terms. As it turned out, refusing to negotiate is common practice that indicates, in the context of accepted Lebanese norms, not a desire to withdraw from the deal, but rather a seriousness of purpose. We can find many cases of multicultural and international stereotypes. That said, the intention here isn't to provide a complete picture, but simply to highlight the relevance of the topic by giving some examples presented through an eight-dimension prism.

1. *Negotiation goal.* In some cultures, the goal of a negotiation is to seal the deal, while for others it's to establish a relationship. Asian negotiators, whose often strive for the latter, tend to spend more time and effort on preliminaries, while North Americans often want to rush through this first phase of deal making.
2. *Willingness to collaborate.* Beyond the given mandate, some negotiators may be more oriented toward working together to come to an agreement. For example, whereas Japanese tend to see negotiations as a collaborative process, this is not the case in western cultures.
3. *Formality.* The level of formality varies from culture to culture. For example, Italians and Germans have a more formal style than North Americans.
4. *Communication style.* In a culture that values directness, such as in North America or Israel, you can expect to receive clear feedback and straightforward answers to your proposals and questions. In cultures based on indirect communication style, as we would find in Japan, you can understand their reaction to your proposals by interpreting seemingly vague comments, gestures, and other signs. Asian negotiators usually adhere to Confucianism, which highly prizes consensus and peaceful communication.
5. *Sensitivity to time.* It is said that Germans are punctual, Mediterranean people are habitually late, Japanese tend to negotiate slowly, while North Americans try to reduce formalities to a minimum and get down to business quickly. Japanese and other Asians, whose goal is to create a relationship rather than simply to sign a contract, need to invest time in the negotiating process.
6. *Emotionalism.* Japanese and many other Asian cultures are inclined to hide their feelings, while Latin Americans and Spaniards tend to show their emotions when negotiating. In the European culture on the whole, Germans and English seem to rank lowest in terms of showing their emotions.
7. *Form of agreement.* Some cultures (such as the Chinese) prefer to draw up a contract initially in the form of general principles and then enumerate all the conditions; others (e.g., North Americans) for the most part prefer

very detailed contracts aiming to anticipate all possible circumstances. In other words, some cultures (e.g., French, Argentinean, Indian) would frame a negotiation as a process that goes from general principles to details, while other cultures (e.g., Japanese, Mexican, Brazilian), from details to general principles.
8. *Team organization.* When negotiating in teams, there may be some cultural differences. In team-based negotiations, e.g., North American, Brazilian, Chinese and Mexican cultures prefer a one-person leadership model. Other cultures (e.g., Japanese) would opt for a consensus-based model.

6.4 HOW TO PREPARE FOR MULTICULTURAL AND INTERNATIONAL NEGOTIATIONS

Like any negotiation, multicultural and international negotiations require thorough preparation, including careful information gathering and analysis. In addition to general recommendations for effective preparation (Chapter 2), this section highlights some specific suggestions for multicultural and international negotiation settings.

It's crucial to avoid the use of stereotypes. As discussed earlier, stereotypes often fail to reflect reality. Relying on them can lead to serious mistakes; for example, assuming that a particular culture inherently operates at a slower pace. Additionally, the use of stereotypes can deeply offend the other party, as they are often exaggerated or presented in a humorous, hyperbolic manner. Morevoer, we need to understand the other party in terms of their cultural identity, recognizing their connection to their country and its values. We should approach each negotiation with an open mind, avoiding assumptions and striving to understand the nuances of the other party's unique perspective. Therefore, we recommend doing a serious analysis and familiarizing yourself with the real traditions that make up the negotiator's cultural identity (not stereotypical ones). If need be, you should learn the customary procedure in the country for conducting meetings.

By understanding and respecting communication styles, etiquette and norms of both everyday life and business and institutional contexts, you can interpret signals correctly and demonstrate respect for the other party's values and practices. For instance, it's useful to strike the appropriate balance between discussing business matters and engaging in more informal conversation, such as talking about family, travel, or personal interests. But be aware that such "small talk" may or may not be considered appropriate, depending on the culture. Understanding your own culture holds the same importance as learning about the culture of the other party. Self-reflection is essential for identifying your cultural identity and values, as well as becoming aware of how they may be perceived by the other party. This awareness helps ensure that cultural differences do not create division but instead foster mutual understanding and respect.

In his book *Negotiating Life* (2013), Jeswald Salacuse describes three ways to address and bridge cultural differences:

1. Adopt the other party's culture and, if possible, align your approach with their norms and practices.
2. Present your own culture positively, showcasing it in a friendly and accommodating manner. For example, during international negotiations, when the other party visits your country, you can organize a cultural program to showcase the achievements of your country.
3. Utilize a third culture. For instance, if people from Portugal and Finland are engaged in negotiations, and they discover they've studied in New Zealand, they can bond over their shared memories.

In general, the most critical aspect of multicultural and international negotiations is the need to respect the other side in terms of their culture, traditions, and ways of doing business. This respect for the differences that may exist, combined with curiosity and a commitment to understanding the other party's perspectives, will create foundation for effective and harmonious negotiations.

In the next chapter, we'll look at how negotiating plays out in the phygital world.

SURVEY
After reading this chapter, think again about the various dimensions that may impact the effectiveness of a multicultural and international negotiation. Have your perspectives shifted?

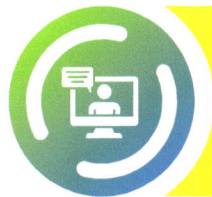

VIDEO INTERVIEWS
What are the most frequent cultural differences you may encounter during negotiations? Find the answer to this and other questions in the next series of interviews with experts.

DIARY
Please take a moment to fill in your personal diary with your key takeaways.

READINGS
Here's a list of resources to help you learn more about this chapter's topics.

SUMMARY

MULTICULTURALISM — Multiculturalism is the existence of many cultures, traditions, habits, peculiarities. Essentially, it gives rise to the need to collaborate with individuals from various cultural backgrounds. We encounter multiculturalism not only when negotiating with representatives from other countries, but also within nations, when we work in multicultural teams and appreciate the richness of diverse cultures.

INTERNATIONALITY — Internationality refers to strengthening international cooperation and unity between different cultures and peoples. Internationality to some extent also includes multiculturalism.

STEREOTYPES — Cultural and national stereotypes refer to widely accepted beliefs that a certain group of people (who share a hometown, home country, or some social attribute, for example) have a certain set of common behavioral features. In fact, stereotyping is a cognitive process of categorization which gives rise to general attitudes toward a specific group of people.

GLOBE CULTURAL DIMENSIONS — The GLOBE identifies nine cultural dimensions that help to explain the differences in values, behaviors, and practices across various cultures.
1. Uncertainty avoidance
2. Power distance
3. Societal collectivism
4. In-group collectivism
5. Gender egalitarianism
6. Assertiveness
7. Future orientation
8. Performance orientation
9. Humane orientation

BARRIERS	• Language • Diverse interpretation of gestures, emotions, and behaviors • Technical • Technological • Gastronomical • Etiquette
EIGHT-DIMENSION PRISM TO PRESENT STEREOTYPED MULTICULTURAL/ INTERNATIONAL NEGOTIATION EXAMPLES	1. Negotiation goal 2. Willingness to collaborate 3. Formality 4. Communication style 5. Sensitivity to time 6. Emotionalism 7. Form of agreement 8. Team organization
HOW TO PREPARE FOR MULTICULTURAL/ INTERNATIONAL NEGOTIATIONS	• Avoid the use of stereotypes. • Understand the other party in terms of their cultural identity. • Understand your own culture. • Respect any differences.

NOTES

[1] Geert Hofstede, "Empirical Models of Cultural Differences," in *Contemporary Issues in Cross-Cultural Psychology*, ed. Nico Bleichrodt and Pieter J. D. Drenth (Swets & Zeitlinger Publishers, 1991), 4–20.

[2] Robert House et al., "Understanding Cultures and Implicit Leadership Theories across the Globe: An Introduction to Project GLOBE," *Journal of World Business* 37, no. 1 (March 2002): 3–10. https://doi.org/10.1016/s1090-9516(01)00069-4.

[3] Ibid., 5.

[4] Ibid., 5.

[5] Ibid., 5.

[6] Ibid., 5.

[7] Ibid., 5.

[8] Ibid., 6.

[9] Ibid., 6.

[10] Ibid., 6.

[11] Ibid., 6.

"We can only see a short distance ahead, but we can see plenty there that needs to be done."

_ALAN TURING

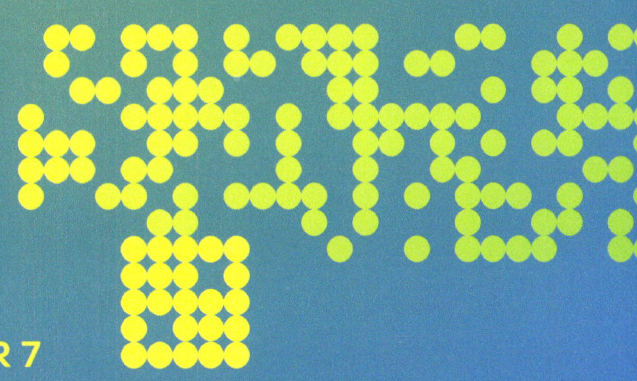

CHAPTER 7

NEGOTIATION IN THE PHYGITAL WORLD

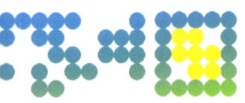

HOW IT WORKS

This chapter explores the art of negotiation in the contemporary "phygital" world, examining how the digital dimension reshapes the dynamics of the negotiation process and offering insights on how to achieve an optimal balance between physical and digital interactions. Additionally, risks and challenges with this hybrid approach are highlighted and strategies to navigate and mitigate them effectively are outlined.
In the following chapter, there are off-line and online activities, such as reading and working on interactive content (survey questions, video interviews, and a personal diary). Below, you'll find detailed instructions on how to engage with this chapter of the book.

SURVEY
To start out this chapter, you'll be given a survey question to help you reflect on the most relevant challenges of phygital negotiations.

7.1 WHAT IS PHYGITAL NEGOTIATION?

Here we'll discuss what phygital negotiation is, how it works, and why it's important to balance traditional and online formats to come up with the ideal recipe. Like everything, this format has advantages and disadvantages. This section addresses the need for adaptability and flexibility, and the ways to overcome risks and challenges such as communication barriers, security issues, and psychological overload.

7.2 HOW PHYGITAL NEGOTIATION WORKS

Here we'll talk about invaluable sets of tools and the peculiarities that come up when you use them while negotiating.

7.3 FUTURE TRENDS OF PHYGITAL NEGOTIATION

Now we'll look into the future and discuss how the further development of technology (such as AR, VR, and AI) can transform the negotiation process.

SURVEY
After reading the chapter, answer the same question about the most relevant challenges of phygital negotiation so you can see how your initial point of view has evolved.

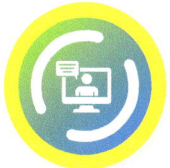

VIDEO INTERVIEWS
In this series of video interviews, we ask experts to share their views on how to overcome the challenges of phygital negotiations and avoid potential traps.

DIARY
Please take a moment to fill in your personal diary with your key takeaways.

READINGS
Here's a list of resources to help you learn more about this chapter's topics.

SUMMARY

SURVEY
Before reading this chapter, think about the elements that may represent a challenge in phygital negotiations and how much they can hinder effective communication.

7.1 WHAT IS PHYGITAL NEGOTIATION?

Phygital negotiation refers to a blend of traditional face-to-face and digital-enabled interactions. In fact, digital tools can enhance the negotiation process in both in-person interactions (with data mining, for instance) and virtual ones (online meetings). In essence, phygital negotiations encompass a wide variety of combinations of direct, personal contacts and technology-driven elements such as online collaboration platforms, data collection and analysis tools, and document sharing systems.

We are already living the phygital world, where communication between people happens through a blend of off-line and online interactions. Technologies are continuously and rapidly evolving, reshaping the way we interact and unlocking opportunities for new forms of integration between digitally-enabled and in-person communication. This integration is also influencing negotiation dynamics. As a result, the skills needed to negotiate in these hybrid contexts are now essential for the modern negotiator.

Phygital negotiation is a multifaced phenomenon. Basically, it refers to the use of a wide range of interaction methods, both in-person and digitally enabled, such as video conferencing, collaborative platforms, technology for document sharing, live messaging systems, tools for data collection and analysis, and AI-powered systems for decision-making processes. Negotiations might take place face-to-face, but the preparatory process (e.g., document sharing, compiling scenarios, follow-up) can be handled digitally.

The following situation represents a simple example of a phygital negotiation. Recently, a negotiation process was completed by two agents located in different countries. They initially met in-person to discuss the possibility of cooperation; this was essential for building trust and rapport. The next stages of the negotiation were conducted through video conference systems; documents were exchanged through cloud-based technologies, and the final agreement was signed thanks to a secure, online digital platform.

Overall, the success of negotiations in the phygital world depends a great deal on a deep understanding and a thoughtful balance between face-to-face (live) and online interactions (whether synchronous or not), and a careful analysis of each unique negotiation situation.

In general, the higher the level of complexity of the negotiation, the more effective live (possibly in-person) interactions are. Let's consider a negotiation between an Italian and an Argentine company. On the Italian side, we have Laura, and on the Argentine side, Andrea. They're discussing shipment details. It's not their first meeting, and so far they've negotiated in-person using a very collaborative approach. Laura keeps asking for another face-to-face meeting, but Andrea doesn't see the need at this stage. Andrea says it's not worth the 18-hour trip, and she's getting a bit frustrated and irritated with Laura's request. This is a classic example where phygital negotiation can satisfy the needs of all the parties involved, ensuring effective interaction.

7.1.1 Advantages and challenges of phygital negotiation

Phygital negotiation provides great flexibility in a variety of circumstances. But at the same time, some risks can emerge.

So far, online negotiations (whether synchronous or not) have offered several distinct advantages, such as breaking down geographical barriers and facilitating interactions between people located in different locations. Additionally, the online component of phygital negotiations offers significant savings in time, cost, and effort, eliminating the need for business trips, flights, accommodation, and other travel-related expenses. The online format is also convenient because it allows parties to engage without being tied to a specific location. Moreover, technology enables the use of shared platforms for cooperation, making it easier to work together seamlessly and efficiently.

However, there are certain challenges associated with the online format in phygital negotiations. For instance, whether or not they are synchronous, online negotiations rely on technologies; any technical problems (such as internet connection issues) can dramatically disrupt the negotiation process. The lack (or low level) of personal interaction may represent another significant risk of online negotiations. Without being able to observe body language, facial expressions, and other non-verbal signs, it's tricky to understand people's emotions and gauge their energy. (See Chapter 4 where we discuss the role of emotions in negotiation.) This can make it harder to establish trust and develop personal relationships.

For example, let's consider a negotiation process between two companies, A and B. The negotiator for A sends an email to the negotiator from B outlining the basic conditions of the negotiation. The message is clearly formulated and straightforward, although lacking any emotion. This tone may be perceived by the negotiator from company B as insufficiently respectful, too harsh. To prevent such situations, it's a good idea to complement your email with a video meeting, allowing the other party in the negotiation to pick up on your emotions, body language, and tone. In any case, it is highly recommended to conduct particularly critical negotiations in-person, as your physical presence will add depth and impact to the interaction.

Face-to-face meetings also eliminate many of the distractions that can arise in online settings, such as household tasks, background noise, or technological interruptions. For example, during an important video meeting, one of the negotiators may have problems with their internet connection. This interruption can cause a negative impression, or annoy the other party, as they'll have to postpone the meeting or wait for the connection to be fixed. So it's important to prepare in advance and have a contingency plan for technology fails.

Although technologies are available and can be used properly even during in-person interactions, in this context there are fewer digital distractions; it's less tempting to check messages or switch tasks, which happens more frequently in online meetings. Furthermore, we should also consider the cultural aspect here too. In fact, in some cultures, such as Middle Eastern countries, face-to-face interaction is highly valued; in others, digital communication is more acceptable, for example, in Scandinavian countries. (See Chapter 6 for more on cultural issues in negotiations.)

It is also meaningful to consider the specificities of the digital tools we would use in phygital negotiation. For instance, email communication has its own distinct characteristics. In email-based negotiations, parties tend to be more wary, often carefully choosing every word they write. This can lead to a more reserved and cautious tone, with negotiators being less open and transparent compared to other forms of communication.

It's worthwhile noting that when using technology, the risk of digital fatigue is high. A simple recommendation to overcome this risk is to plan breaks and set time limits for online meetings. Other than digital fatigue, over-reliance on technology can lead to a deterioration of the relationship between the negotiators; neglecting live interactions (be they online or in-person) will ultimately erode the effectiveness of negotiations.

Security plays a vital role when technology is used in negotiations. In phygital negotiations there is a critical question about data protection and confidentiality. At present, any cyberattacks or leaks in negotiation information can result in the loss of a competitive advantage and may even lead to ethical, reputational, business and legal issues. Some basic approaches to mitigate these risks should be established, such as selecting online tools with robust security features; ensuring strong password protection; implementing clear security protocols; and providing thorough training for negotiators.

Building trust represents a top challenge for negotiators in a phygital context. When possible, negotiators should prioritize real-time communications, such as video calls, which help to foster more effective, transparent interaction. However, the principle of transparency must be applied in both the digital and physical dimensions, ensuring that openness and clarity are maintained throughout the negotiation process, regardless of the medium.

7.2 HOW PHYGITAL NEGOTIATION WORKS

A phygital negotiation is a highly demanding and complex process, so as with any type of negotiation, planning and thoughtful preparation are key. It's not enough to simply blend in-person and online modes; instead, it's crucial to create a cohesive model that effectively integrates both into a unified process. For example, videoconferencing might be applied to connect global participants, while taking a traditional face-to-face approach for local stakeholders' meetings. This ensures a seamless experience that accommodates the unique needs of all the parties involved.

When preparing a phygital negotiation, the critical step is to choose the most appropriate digital tools. A wide range of such tools is available, designed to foster negotiation, encourage teamwork, and enable seamless document sharing, instant data exchanges, and a real-time communication process. These tools help cultivate a strong sense of "presence," even when people are working remotely.

Among the most essential and widely used negotiation tools, several distinct categories can be identified. We would like to emphasize that our aim is not to promote any specific tool or platform, but rather to describe the key categories of tools that support negotiations and provide some examples.

Platforms for supporting virtual meetings and interactions allow negotiations through video conferencing systems with the possibility of automatic transcriptions, a whiteboard for brainstorming and discussions, the creation of surveys and other interactive elements during meetings and presentations (e.g., Bambook, Miro, Mentimeter, Microsoft Teams, Zoom, Google Meet, Cisco WebEx). For example, a clothing retailer may want to negotiate with several companies located in different countries at the same time to discuss the details of multiple new store openings.

Collaboration platforms allow people to work together on files and share them while conducting video calls; such platforms also provide access to project management tools that can be integrated with other services and communication systems (e.g., Slack, Trello, Asana). For example, let's take a complex negotiation with a large number of resources on the table. In this case, a digital tool can be used which allows participants to create separate channels to efficiently discuss specific resources or items (such as prices, logistics, marketing, or service). Then they can bring in the other stakeholders as need be.

To co-create and manage documents, there are cloud-based systems which make it possible to share files with all parties, even allowing them to work on these documents in real time (e.g., Google Drive, Microsoft OneDrive). There are also services that enable digital signatures, for instance such tools as Zoho Sign, Signeasy, Docusign, and e.Signatures.io. If authorized by law and accepted in organizational policies, these services save considerable time and reduce bureaucracy, as they eliminate the need to gather signatures from multiple parties over an extended period.

Other simpler tools also exist, such as WhatsApp or WeChat, which allow teams to keep in touch (by sending group messages, sharing announcements, and so forth), facilitating quick and efficient communication updates.

Many AI-based systems are already available, and there are many more to come. These systems offer an extensive range of high-speed capabilities.

They are able to compile a negotiation schedule; prepare a formal presentation; draft an email; take the minutes from a meeting; support the profiling of negotiating parties and even help to recognize their emotions (e.g., Kira Systems, Crystal, Cogito); analyze large quantity of data on market trends, economic conditions, company performance, and negotiation dynamics; and formulate multiple trajectories and trends, empowering predictive capacity, and enabling data-driven decisions.

Moreover, AI-based tools can simulate live negotiation meetings, emulating human behavior in different scenarios (Sedric is one), so we can practice our own negotiation skills. The AI Negotiation Advisor (AINA) aims to be a concrete application of AI-based systems in negotiations. AINA can listen to the negotiation dialogue in real-time, analyze it through models and frameworks of reference, and suggest the next move the negotiator should make.

7.3 FUTURE TRENDS OF PHYGITAL NEGOTIATION

There is an ongoing debate about the future development of the phygital world in general, and phygital negotiations in particular. The most radical analysts predict that one of the components – either online or in-person – will eventually come to dominate. But opinions vary, with some believing that physical contact will make a strong comeback, and others arguing that the shift towards online spaces will only intensify. However, most researchers agree that the coexistence of online and in-person elements will continue. At the same time, they acknowledge that certain trends will dramatically shape the future of the negotiation landscape.

Researchers and practitioners recognize the profound impact of innovation on the future of negotiations. One of the most significant is the exponential rise in the power of data analytics. Increasingly, negotiations will be driven by fast collection and analysis of big data, and sophisticated data-driven prediction models and decision-making processes. For instance, let's take a company in the tourism industry, and say that Sally, a team member of the marketing department, intends to propose a new product to the head of her department. In other words, Sally has to negotiate with her team manager. To prepare, she can gauge consumer reactions to her proposal by aggregating digital footprints, such as reviews from platforms like TripAdvisor. By gathering hundreds of thousands of reviews (together with other analysis), Sally can prepare a strong case for the new product, and allow her team manager to take a robust, informed decision.

The development of virtual and augmented reality represents a key innovation which is shaping the negotiation landscape. For example, through virtual reality, it is now possible to showcase a product that has yet to be rolled out or to simulate a service that's still in the design phase. This can enhance the presentation of new ideas in a highly immersive and interactive way. Additionally, virtual and augmented reality can compensate for some of the limitations of modern online negotiation.

Advances in the Internet of Things, machine learning and above all artificial intelligence (AI) are predicted to be among the most influential factors in the transformation of negotiations. While it's difficult to predict the exact trajectory of AI, its growth is already rapid, and many tasks currently performed by negotiators can be successfully carried out by AI. This shift will fundamentally transform the negotiation process, making it more data-driven and efficient at the very least, and hopefully more effective as well.

Emotional and psychological dimensions are highly influential aspects in the evolution of phygital negotiations. Currently, we have not made much progress in understanding how perceptions and emotions differ in either physical, digital, or phygital formats. Grasping the relevant nuances is vital for future negotiations in order to tailor approaches accordingly.

As we know, culture has a powerful influence in negotiations, and this is also true in the context of the phygital space. In fact, there is a common misconception that cultural sensitivity is diminished in phygital negotiation, but this does not seem to be the case. Future developments of phygital negotiation should focus on more in-depth research and greater attention to cultural sensitivity. This will be key to fostering more effective and inclusive phygital negotiations.

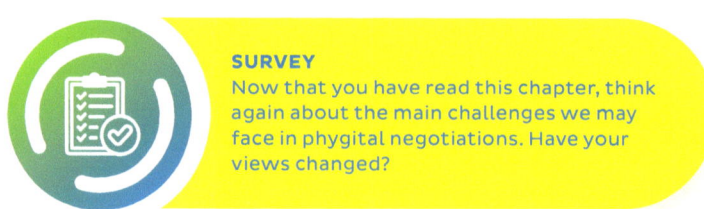

SURVEY
Now that you have read this chapter, think again about the main challenges we may face in phygital negotiations. Have your views changed?

CHAPTER 7 | NEGOTIATION IN THE PHYGITAL WORLD

VIDEO INTERVIEWS
In this series of video interviews, we ask experts to share their insights on how to overcome the challenges in phygital negotiations and avoid potential traps.

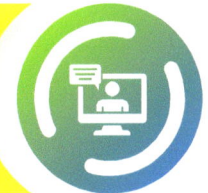

DIARY
Please take a moment to fill in your personal diary with your key takeaways.

READINGS
Here's a list of resources to help you learn more about this chapter's topics.

SUMMARY

PHYGITAL NEGOTIATION	This refers to the use of a wide range of interaction methods, both in-person and digitally-enabled. Overall, the success of negotiations in the phygital world is contingent on a deep understanding and a thoughtful balance between face-to-face (that is, live) and online interactions (synchronous or not), and a careful analysis of each unique negotiation situation.
ADVANTAGES AND DISADVANTAGES	• High level of adaptability and flexibility • Increase of efficiency • Communication barriers • Over-reliance on technology • Security and privacy issues • Establishment of trust
CATEGORIES OF DIGITAL TOOLS	• Platforms for supporting virtual meetings and interactions • Collaboration platforms • Systems for co-creating and managing documents • Digital signatures • AI-based systems
HOW TO NAVIGATE PHYGITAL NEGOTIATION	• Be prepared. • Overcome communication barriers. • Mitigate risks. • Do not overly rely on technology. • Pay attention to security issues. • Build trust.

FUTURE TRENDS OF PHYGITAL NEGOTIATION

- Innovation will shape the future of negotiations.
- Negotiations will be driven by collecting and analyzing big data, and by using sophisticated data-driven prediction models and decision-making processes.
- The development of virtual and augmented reality will impact negotiations.
- Advances in artificial intelligence are predicted to be one of the most influential factors.
- We'll see more systematic integration of physical and digital elements.
- Cybersecurity and privacy with regard to personal and sensitive data will emerge as important trends.
- We'll have a greater awareness and understanding of the relative emotional, psychological, and cultural dimensions.

DIGITAL TOOLS

WORD CLOUD
This tool lets you input keywords on a topic and shows the most common words, adjusting their size and color based on frequency.

SURVEY
These questionnaires collect your opinions on different topics and let you compare your responses with those of other readers.

VIDEO INTERVIEWS
Interviews with experts provide an interactive learning experience, including questions to enhance your understanding.

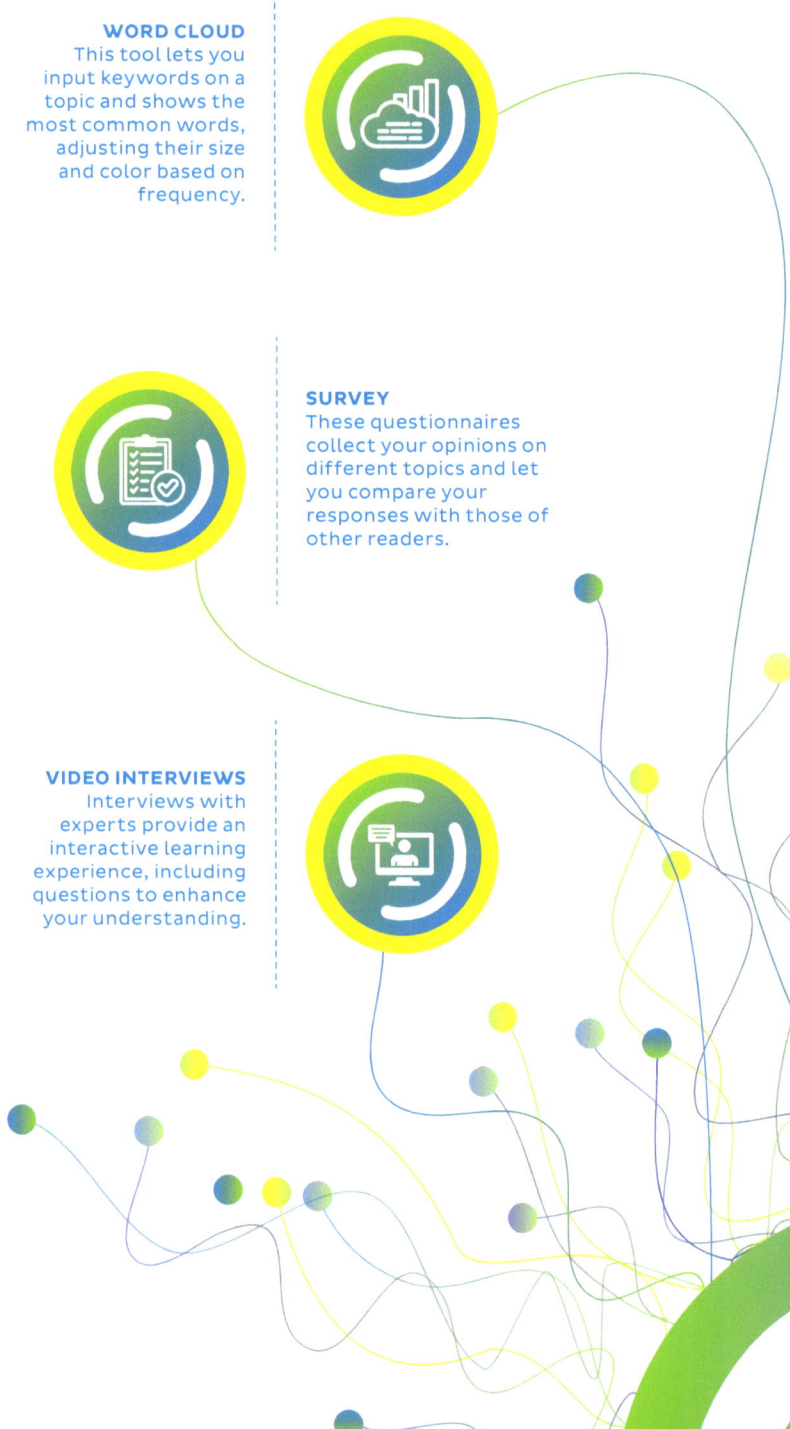

SELF-ASSESSMENT
These tests help you discover more about yourself by offering an initial assessment and identifying areas for improvement.

SELF-REFLECTION QUESTIONS
These questions are usually asked twice to allow you to compare your answers and see how your ideas have changed.

DIARY
We invite you to fill in your diary and review what you have read, leaving your key ideas, questions, and notes for further reflection.

**Fold open and look inside
to discover the contents of this book,
including digital tools!**

To access the digital version, go to
https://digitabook.egeaonline.it and register.
Once logged in, enter the following code:

4473LXRNuk

www.ingramcontent.com/pod-product-compliance
Lightning Source LLC
Chambersburg PA
CBHW040218220526
45473CB00001B/38